Roundworms - A Survey From Past to Present

Edited by Nihal Dogan

Published in London, United Kingdom

Roundworms - A Survey From Past to Present
http://dx.doi.org/10.5772/intechopen.102153
Edited by Nihal Dogan

Contributors
Charles D. Mackenzie, Wilfred L. Mandara, Esther Mwakitalu, Solomon Tadesse, Eyael Tewelde, Parvaiz Yousuf, Semran Parvaiz, Shahid Razzak, Nisheet Zehbi, Narendra Nath Mukhopadhyay, Nihal Dogan

First published in London, United Kingdom, 2023 by IntechOpen
IntechOpen is the global imprint of INTECHOPEN LIMITED, registered in England and Wales, registration number: 11086078, 5 Princes Gate Court, London, SW7 2QJ, United Kingdom

British Library Cataloguing-in-Publication Data
A catalogue record for this book is available from the British Library

Additional hard and PDF copies can be obtained from orders@intechopen.com

Roundworms - A Survey From Past to Present
Edited by Nihal Dogan
p. cm.
Print ISBN 978-1-80356-713-6
Online ISBN 978-1-80356-714-3
eBook (PDF) ISBN 978-1-80356-715-0

Meet the editor

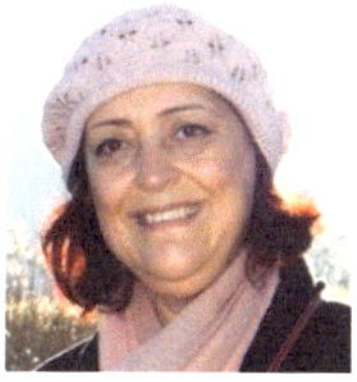

Prof. Dr. Nihal Dogan has worked in the Department of Microbiology at the Faculty of Medicine, Osmangazi University, since 1986. Her master's and Ph.D. thesis focused on the diagnosis and seroepidemiology of *Toxoplasmosis*. She was a visiting researcher on the diagnosis of *Entamoeba histolytica* at the University of Virginia in 2003 and an observer researcher at the Universidad De Chile Faculty of Medicine in 2016, working on *Trypanosomes*. She was appointed a professor in 2008 and is the leading academic in the field of parasitology, with expertise in the epidemiology of parasitic diseases. Her research interests include medical ethics, seroepidemiological survey, intestinal, blood, tissue, and ocular parasites, vector-borne diseases, and zoonotic parasites. Her research has been published in more than 40 national and international journals. She also made 85 poster presentations, plus many oral presentations and keynote speeches at international and national congresses. She has written numerous book chapters on infectious diseases, clinical parasitology, clinical microbiology, and medical microbiology laboratory applications and manuals.

Contents

Preface

The phylum *Nematoda*, also known as roundworms, has more than 30,000 members and is one of the oldest disease-causing creatures of civilization, having been recorded as far back as ancient Greece and Rome. Nematodes consist of three classes, eight subclasses, 12 super-orders, 32 orders, 53 suborders, 101 super-families, 276 families, 511 subfamilies, 3030 genera and 28537 species. They inhabit different environments, with a significant number living as parasites in various human tissues and organs. Parasitic diseases caused by intestinal and tissue nematodes are an important cause of morbidity and mortality across the world, especially in children. They are most frequently seen in countries where clean water supply and sanitation are lacking. Some roundworms (such as *Ascaris, Strongyloides*, and hookworms) can be transmitted through contaminated soil, while others are transmitted to humans through a vector (filarial nematodes). Adult nematodes of other species living in our immediate environment (*Toxocara, Drophilaria*) can also cause zoonotic larva migrans disease in humans.

A quarter of the world's population, mainly in developing countries, is reported to be exposed to soil-borne roundworms. Some roundworms are vector-borne and cause different pathologies in the eye, subcutaneous connective tissue and lymphatic system, called filarial nematode infections. Eight important species of filarial nematodes live in the blood and lymphatic system and cause elephantiasis in humans. It is estimated that more than 120,000 people in tropical countries are infected with filarial nematodes, which are almost impossible to treat. Despite the various measures taken today, it is estimated that only half of the people living in at-risk areas are diagnosed and treated. In this book, the historical development of some nematodes parasitizing humans, their morphological structures, transmission routes, and pathogenic properties are discussed. The topics included are defined by the keywords *Ascaris lumbricoides*, *Enterobius vermicularis*, *Trichuris trichiura*, hookworm, *Strongyloides stercoralis*, filarial nematodes, *Wuchereria bancrofti, Bruggia malayi, Onchocerca volvulus*, larva migrans diseases, and paleoparasitology.

Dr. Nihal Dogan
Professor,
Faculty of Medicine,
Department of Microbiology,
Eskisehir Osmangazi University,
Eskisehir, Turkey

Chapter 1

Introductory Chapter: Roundworms from Past to Present

Nihal Dogan

1. Introduction

More than 30,000 members of the phylum Nematoda, also known as roundworms, live in different habitats. This number increases even more with phylogenetic studies [1, 2].

Some of these are free-living organisms in terrestrial and aquatic environments. A significant number are parasitic on animals and plants. Their bodies are bilaterally symmetrical, without segments, covered with a cuticle layer. They are separate sexes, but there are rare hermaphrodite species. The first nematode identified in humans was Ascaris, described by Linneaus in 1758. Classification studies started in 1808 when Rudolphin used the name "Nematoidea." Various types of phylogenetic research on nematode systematics are carried out by continuously changing molecular techniques. These studies have added many new species to the nematode group [1–3].

Phylum Nematoda: based on evolutionary relationships, developmental and morphological features and recent molecular evidence, a new classification model was created in 2019. Accordingly, Nematodas consist of three classes, eight subclasses, 12 superorders, 32 orders, 53 suborders, 101 superfamilies, 276 families, 511 subfamilies, 3030 genera and 28,537 species [1].

Nematode diseases are one of the oldest diseases of civilization, having been recited as far back as ancient Greece and Rome. The many of hookworms, whipworms or flamentous worms are also called soilborn worms. The many of hookworms, whipworms or flamentous worms are also called soilborn worms. They are more common in children and women and cause intestinal disorders, growth and development disorders, cognitive impairment and death [4].

It is estimated that a quarter of the world's population is infected with soil-transmitted nematodes such as hookworms, Ascaris, Trichuris and Schistosoma. Their presence is still a major cause of morbidity and mortality in developing countries, especially in Africa. According to WHO data, the burden of nematode diseases is greater than that of the world's most common major tropical diseases, such as trypanosomiasis, dengue fever and leprosy [5]. It is estimated that 75% of children in endemic areas are infected and require treatment [5, 6].

Some nematodes are vector-borne and cause different pathologies in the eye, subcutaneous connective tissue and lymphatic system, called filarial nematode infections. Eight important species of filarial nematodes live in the blood and lymph system and cause elephantiasis in humans. Filarial nematodes need a second intermediate host, defined as a vector, to complete their evolution. Their spread worldwide depends on the regions where these intermediate hosts are located. Today, it is known

IntechOpen

that more than 120 thousand people in tropical countries are infected with filarial nematodes. Symptoms of filarial nematode disease include overgrowth of connective tissues due to obstruction of the lymphatic system and consequent overgrowth of the legs, arms, scrotum, vulva and mammary tissues [5–8].

Onchocerciasis, another filarial nematode disease that causes blindness in humans, occurs in the Arabian peninsula, Africa and parts of South and Central America. Transmitted by river flies, Onchocerca and Loa loa cause blindness in more than 37,000 people in endemic areas. *Dirofilaria immitis* (canine heartworm), a zoonotic agent in various countries of the world, especially in the USA, is another common filarial nematode. *Dracunculus medinensis*, which is transmitted through freshwater crustaceans in some parts of Africa where thirst is common, is one of the longest filamentous nematodes common in the world. They are localized in subcutaneous connective tissue [5, 6, 8, 9].

The larval stages of nematodes, whose adult forms live in the intestines of some animals in our immediate environment, cause "*larval migrans*" diseases in humans. It is especially widespread in children who have intensive contact with animals and soil, and in those who come into contact with infected animals. Since the symptoms can be recognized with many other diseases, it is estimated that there are many more cases than known. Although larval nematodes cannot develop into adult form in humans, they can cause severe damage such as hepatosplenomegaly, blindness and death in addition to allergic symptoms. *Toxocariasis* is one of the zoonotic helminth infections with the highest prevalence globally, especially in tropical and rural areas [6, 10–12].

While some nematodes can directly infect and parasitize humans, others may have one or more hosts in their evolution. However, one of their common life traits is that they all go through four different larval stages before they develop into adults. They are usually hermaphroditic and reproduce by eggs. The eggs laid by their hosts in the external environment are found in the soil until they reach a certain maturity, and the temperature and humidity of the soil are essential in their geographical spread. Nematodes with the soil-borne transmission have almost no chance of transmission in regions where the temperature drops below 10°C. However, there are also free-living species in Arctic regions and thermal waters. Approximately 30% of the more than 28,000 species identified to date are known to parasitize marine and freshwater vertebrates [6, 7, 10].

Today, improved sanitation, hygiene education and the widespread use of anthelmintics reduce the disease burden of nematodes. However, both intestinal and vector-borne nematodes remain prevalent in developing countries [5, 6, 10].

In addition to their negative effects on living organisms, nematodes have many significant benefits, such as transforming the ecosystem, directing genetic and toxicity studies, playing an active role in biological warfare, taking part in the food chain and being used in the fight against autoimmune diseases [13].

2. History

Parasites recovered from human remains and mummified human bodies at archeological excavations make an important contribution to the analysis of past lives. For example, Enterobius eggs and lizard parasites, isolated from human bodies dating back to 100,000 BC, indicate that they were feeding on lizards and were in close contact with other primates [14].

Ascaris eggs have been found in organic remains dating back 30,000 years. Another prehistoric study showed that Ascaris were widespread among both South and North American Indians. Archeologists suggest that they spread here after migrations from the old world. Nematodes such as hookworms and Tirichuris date back 9000 years. Paleoparasitological studies have also shown that soil-borne nematodes, which are common in Africa and Europe, arrived in the Americas much later [3, 4, 14].

Historians have learned from genome studies of coprological materials that parasitic infections accompanied the evolution of humans. In this way, much has been revealed about the origin of man. From this information, we learn that the first humans emerged as *Homo sapiens* about 150 thousand years ago in East Africa and spread around the world in waves. During their migrations, they brought some parasites with them and collected some of them from the roads and spread across the globe with their parasites. In this spread, contact with soil during agricultural practices and contact with animals have also been factors that facilitate transmission. The formation of cities and increased human density were other factors that facilitated transmission. In the 1500s, with the opening of the slave trade and other trade routes to the world, endemic species spread to other continents [14–17].

In paleoparasitological studies, hookworms were identified in Africa around 7000 BC. As with other helminths, they are estimated to have spread to the Americas in the following years through the slave trade. During these investigations, examining naturally or artificially fossilized coprolites and tissue samples helps us define the history of parasites and human evolution [14, 18].

The first written records date back to Egyptian papyrus between 3000 and 400 BC. Later, parasites were described in the works of the ancient Greek physician Hippocrates. Diseases caused by parasites were mentioned in Chinese medicine between 3000 and 300 BC, in India in 2500–200, in Rome in 700 BC and 400 AD and by Arab physicians in 850–953 AD. This was a period when medieval Europe was inadequate in science due to religion and superstition, but with the renaissance, great discoveries began in the nineteenth century with Pastor, Koch, Roux and Manson [12, 16].

Ascaris was the first nematode to be identified in mummies. One of the best-documented parasitic diseases known from the earliest times was Dracunculus medinensis, a parasite up to 80 cm in length living in subcutaneous connective tissue. It was mentioned in the Eber papyrus in 1500 BC. It has been shown on Egyptian mummies. It was described as a febrile snake disease that enveloped the Red Sea. It is also mentioned in the Bible and the book was written by Arab physicians in the seventh century BC [4, 14, 17].

Nematodes are among the oldest known parasitic diseases of mankind. Ascaris was mentioned by physicians in ancient Greece and Rome. Since the late nineteenth century, they have been the subject of important scientific studies. For example, meiosis and gametogenesis, the basis of chromosome studies, were carried out on Ascaris species. They are expected to form the basis of future molecular and genomic studies of biological processes [4, 18, 19].

Filarial worms were described by Manson in 1877. Historically, lymphatic filariasis was widespread along the Nile River, as evidenced by the swollen limbs of a statue dating from 2000 BC. In the sixteenth century, the disease was described as the curse of St. Thomas. However, it was not until after the microscope's discovery that the disease's larval stage was elucidated [3, 4].

Hookworms were described in general terms by Tyson in 1683. In 1836, the dermal transmission of hookworm larvae was described after a laboratory accident [20].

In Utah, North America, *Enterobius vermicularis* eggs have been isolated from caves inhabited by settlers 10,000 years ago. This represents the oldest human parasite isolated from coprolites in 7837 BC. In Asia, *E. vermicularis* eggs were found in a 7000-year-old female skeleton in Iran, representing the presence of the infection on this continent [14, 16, 17].

After the 2000s, the rates of *Ascaris* and *Trichuris*, the most common intestinal nematodes worldwide, have decreased by 10% with various measures and preventive medication. However, the numbers are still high. Almost all nematode infections are diseases of poverty. All living things, especially humans, are at risk in places where there is no clean food and water and where sanitation is inadequate [21–23].

3. Diagnosis

Hundreds of millions of people worldwide, especially in developing countries, live with intestinal and tissue nematodes. In recent years, the spread of nematodes from endemic areas to different countries has increased due to wars, migration and tourist travel. Despite the various technological possibilities in developed countries, there are difficulties in diagnosis due to problems in diagnosis. Parasitologic diagnosis is often difficult to obtain, while serologic diagnosis is less reliable due to cross-reactions between helminth species. Molecular tests are not ubiquitous and still need optimization [22–24].

Laboratory diagnosis depends on the location of the nematode in the body. Methods for demonstrating the causative agent are always the gold standard in diagnosis. While the criteria for diagnosis and classification are based on the morphological and morphometric characteristics of the nematode, serological and molecular methods are also used today. Serologic methods can sometimes lead to misdiagnosis due to the common cuticle antigen of nematodes. Molecular methods are very successful in species identification and phylogenetic studies, but they can only be applied in certain research centres and are time-consuming. MALDI-TOF, a new identification method, is based on detecting particles released after ionization of samples with a laser [22]. Studying the protein profiles of pathogenic nematodes with this method can help decipher host-pathogen interactions [5, 6, 18, 22, 24–26].

4. Results

WHO recommends microscopic examination using the Kato-Katz method to diagnose soil-transmitted nematodes. The sedimentation technique has been found to be more successful in preparing stool samples. Intestinal obstructions require urgent surgery. In endemic areas, nutritional and vitamin supplements for children alleviate the damage of nematodes. Single-dose chemotherapy, recommended by WHO since 2001, is one of the measures to protect school-age children. Although anthelmintic drugs are available, they do not provide long-term protection against reinfection.

Since 2000, the World Health Organization has launched the Global Program to "Eliminate Lymphatic Filariasis," which affects 863 million people in 47 countries. According to 2018 data, there has been a 74% decrease in the disease rate since the start of the program. Key targets for surveillance and treatment were decided to be maintained beyond 2020.

Despite the measures taken in low-income countries, nematodes still remain the most critical public health problem. Drug resistance emerging in endemic areas reduces success rates in treatment. There is a need to take new steps in the fight against nematodes by reviewing recently developed genetic studies.

Author details

Nihal Dogan
Eskisehir Osmangazi University, Turkey

*Address all correspondence to: nihaldogan42@gmail.com

References

[1] Hodda M. Phylum Nematoda: A classification, catalogue and index of valid genera, with a census of valid species. Zootaxa. 2022;**5114**(1):1-289. DOI: 10.11646/zootaxa.5114.1.110.11646/zootaxa.5114.1.1

[2] Ahmed M, Holovachov O. Twenty years after de ley and blaxter-how far did we progress in understanding the phylogeny of the phylum nematoda? Animals (Basel). 2021;**11**(12):3479. DOI: 10.3390/ani11123479

[3] Blaxter M, Koutsovoulos G. The evolution of parasitism in Nematoda. Parasitology. 2015;**142 Suppl 1** (Suppl. 1):S26-S39. DOI: 10.1017/S0031182014000791

[4] Araújo A, Reinhard K, Ferreira LF, Pucu E, Chieffi PP. Paleoparasitology: The origin of human parasites. Arquivos de Neuro-Psiquiatria. 2013;**71**(9B):722-726. DOI: 10.1590/0004-282X20130159

[5] WHO. Reducing Risks, Promoting Healthy Life. The World Health Report 2002. Geneva: World Health Organization; 2002. p. 192. Annex Table 3. Burden of Disease in DALYs by Cause, Sex and Mortality Stratus in WHO Regions, Estimates for 2001

[6] Broker S, Michael E. The potential of geographical information systems and remote sensing in the epidemiology and control of human helminth infections. Advances in Parasitology. 2000;**47**:245-288. DOI: 10.1016/s0065-308x(00)47011-9

[7] Brooker S. Estimating the global distribution and disease burden of intestinal nematode infections: Adding up the numbers—A review. International Journal for Parasitology. 2010;**40**(10):1137-1144. DOI: 10.1016/j.ijpara.2010.04.004

[8] Available from: https://www.who.int/

[9] Riebenbauer K, Weber PB, Walochnik J, Karlhofer F, Winkler S, Dorfer S, et al. Human dirofilariosis in Austria: The past, the present, the future. Parasites & Vectors. 2021;**14**(1):227. DOI: 10.1186/s13071-021-04696-4

[10] Loukas A, Maizels RM, Hotez PJ. The yin and yang of human soil-transmitted helminth infections. International Journal for Parasitology. 2021;**51**(13-14): 1243-1253. DOI: 10.1016/j.ijpara.2021.11.001

[11] Landmann JK, Prociv P. Experimental human infection with the dog hookworm, Ancylostoma caninum. Medical Journal of Australia. 2003;**178**(2):69-71. DOI: 10.5694/j.1326-5377.2003.tb05222.x

[12] Nicoletti A. Toxocariasis. Handbook of Clinical Neurology. 2013;**114**:217-228. DOI: 10.1016/B978-0-444-53490-3.00016-9

[13] Peters A. Application and commercialization of nematodes. Applied Microbiology and Biotechnology. 2013;**97**(14):6181-6188. DOI: 10.1007/s00253-013-4941-7

[14] Fry GF, Moore JG. Enterobius vermicularis: 10,000-year-old human infection. Science. 1969;**166**(3913):1620. DOI: 10.1126/science.166.3913.1620

[15] Yeates GW, Bongers T, De Goede RG, Freckman DW, Georgieva SS. Feeding habits in soil nematode families and genera—An outline for soil

ecologists. Journal of Nematology. 1993;**25**(3):315-331

[16] Araújo A, Ferreira LF. Oxiuríase e migrações pré-históricas [Oxyuriasis and prehistoric migrations]. Hist Cienc Saude Manguinhos. 1995;**2**(1):99-109. DOI: 10.1590/s0104-59701995000200006

[17] Paknazhad N, Mowlavi G, Dupouy Camet J, Jelodar ME, Mobedi I, Makki M, et al. Paleoparasitological evidence of pinworm (*Enterobius vermicularis*) infection in a female adolescent residing in ancient Tehran (Iran) 7000 years ago. Parasites & Vectors. 2016;**9**:33. DOI: 10.1186/s13071-016-1322-y

[18] Castelletto ML, Gang SS, Hallem EA. Recent advances in functional genomics for parasitic nematodes of mammals. The Journal of Experimental Biology. 2020;**223**(Pt Suppl. 1):jeb206482. DOI: 10.1242/jeb.206482

[19] Crompton DW. Ascaris and ascariasis. Advances in Parasitology. 2001;**48**:285-375. DOI: 10.1016/s0065-308x(01)48008-0

[20] Brooker S, Bethony J, Hotez PJ. Human hookworm infection in the 21st century. Advances in Parasitology. 2004;**58**:197-288. DOI: 10.1016/S0065-308X(04)58004-1

[21] Vercruysse J, Levecke B, Prichard R. Human soil-transmitted helminths: Implications of mass drug administration. Current Opinion in Infectious Diseases. 2012;**25**(6):703-708. DOI: 10.1097/QCO.0b013e328358993a

[22] Seesao Y, Gay M, Merlin S, Viscogliosi E, Aliouat-Denis CM, Audebert C. A review of methods for nematode identification. Journal of Microbiological Methods. 2017;**138**:37-49. DOI: 10.1016/j.mimet.2016.05.030

[23] Mabaso ML, Appleton CC, Hughes JC, Gouws E. The effect of soil type and climate on hookworm (*Necator americanus*) distribution in KwaZulu-Natal, South Africa. Tropical Medicine & International Health. 2003;**8**(8):722-727. DOI: 10.1046/j.1365-3156.2003.01086.x

[24] Northern C, Grove DI. Strongyloides stercoralis: Antigenic analysis of infective larvae and adult worms. International Journal for Parasitology. 1990;**20**(3):381-387. DOI: 10.1016/0020-7519(90)90155-g

[25] Lustigman S, Prichard RK, Gazzinelli A, Grant WN, Boatin BA, McCarthy JS, et al. A research agenda for helminth diseases of humans: The problem of helminthiases. PLoS Neglected Tropical Diseases. 2012;**6**(4):e1582. DOI: 10.1371/journal.pntd.0001582

[26] Chapman PR, Giacomin P, Loukas A, McCarthy JS. Experimental human hookworm infection: A narrative historical review. PLoS Neglected Tropical Diseases. 2021;**15**(12):e0009908. DOI: 10.1371/journal.pntd.0009908

Chapter 2

Understanding the Pathogenesis of the Major Human Filarial Nematode Infections

Charles D. Mackenzie, Wilfred L. Mandara and Esther Mwakitalu

Abstract

Filarial infections are very common across the animal kingdom despite their tendency to be host specific. Although often being silent infections with relatively little clinical consequence, three filarial infections can cause significant morbidity: onchocerciasis (OV) (caused by *Onchocerca volvulus*) and lymphatic filariasis (LF) (caused by *Wuchereria bancrofti* or *Brugia sp*), and in the veterinary world, the common canine condition of dirofilariasis. Successful elimination programs for these have been developed in the endemic countries based on extensive chemotherapy distribution, and these have catalysed a much greater understanding of the treatment and epidemiology of these infections. In contrast, the pathogenesis and clinical presentation of the two human filarial diseases, and a third, loiasis—which can complicate chemotherapy distribution in OV and LF co-endemic areas—are still not well understood. This present discussion addresses recent knowledge concerning the pathogenesis and presentation of the two major human filariases and makes suggestions as to approaches that could be taken to better understand their pathobiology and clinical forms. Better understanding and improved monitoring of the clinical condition are both likely to augment the already successful progress to global elimination.

Keywords: lymphatic filariasis, onchocerciasis, pathogenesis, investigation, assessment

1. Introduction

Nematode infections are complicated and still poorly understood infectious agents. The fact that being large, anatomically and biochemically complex organisms they can still live and multiply within their hosts (**Table 1**), often without any obvious clinical signs and symptoms, reflects a remarkable degree of adaptation they have undergone during their evolution. Filariae are arguably the most extraordinary of the nematode species, which are widely distributed throughout nature in being present in many host species, although are nevertheless often confined to a single host species. It should also be noted that non-filarial nematodes can also be present in their host without obvious external indications—a classical example being *Ascaris sp.* which migrates through the body, arguably through the circulation, without major clinical

Stage/component	Characteristic	Location	
L1	Microfilaria	Host and vector	Identifiable
L2	Intra-vector stage	Vector	Identifiable
L3	Infective stage	Vector and host	Identifiable in vector
L4	Relatively short-lived developing stage	Host- little known	Not identified
L5/Adult	Long lived		Identifiable
Uterine components	Biologically active in the host		Identifiable

Table 1.
Different stages in the development of a filarial nematode.

external signs to the lungs to finally reach the intestine again with a mild cough being the only obvious clinical presentation. However, filariae are parasites that do not just migrate through their host's internal tissues but also mate and multiply within the host's tissues, a biologically complex activity that arguably requires a high level of adaptation, or manipulation, of the host's natural ability to react to and reject foreign materials and substances. This present communication aims to describe recent changes in our understanding and perceptions of the major filarial diseases, and to emphasise that it is important, if there are to be useful advances in the global progress to elimination filarial infections, to better understanding their pathobiology and clinical presentation.

Historically filarial infections have generally been placed in the category of "clinical oddities" and have been commonly known by somewhat emotive titles: "River Blindness" for onchocerciasis, "Calabar Swelling" for loiasis, and "elephantiasis" with LF [1, 2]. All of these titles actually lack accuracy as appropriate descriptors of the actual infections. Onchocerciasis is more commonly a dermatological condition rather than an ophthalmic disease—although the blindness induced in severe cases is undoubtedly clinically significant. Loiasis is known more commonly now as "eye worm"—due to observable passage of the adult worm across the conjunctiva, which is more common than the sub-dermal swellings. Clinically, loiasis is better known for the adverse central nervous system responses that can occur post chemotherapeutic treatment rather than a serious clinical disease in its own right. Use of the term "elephantiasis" for LF is now regarded as being unacceptable in a disease that is associated with high levels of stigma in those affected—comparing this condition to an elephant's skin is not appropriate for either the human, or the innocently defamed elephant. Unfortunately, this condition is already extraordinarily well known across the globe by the term "elephantiasis," as is the image of the dramatic scrotal swelling that occurs due to hydrocoele induced by LF infection. Thus, it is important that we learn more about the characteristics of these diseases through careful observation and operational investigations and that we change old perceptions through dissemination of new data driven by new, well-investigated, information about their pathogenesis, interpretation, and treatment.

Our general understanding of filarial infections today has been largely driven by two major issues—firstly, the search for an effective and safe chemotherapeutic treatment and secondly, the decision that the major two of these groups' human filarial infections, onchocerciasis (*Onchocerca volvulus*) and the lymphatic filariae (*Wuchereria bancrofti* and *Brugia* sp.) could be controlled and subsequently eliminated [3]. The latter of the two by either through interrupting transmission as

DOI: http://dx.doi.org/10.5772/intechopen.106879

with human onchocerciasis, or in the case of human LF by reducing infection and morbidity so that it is no longer a major public health problem [1]. The other filarial nematode that has featured historically in terms of research and clinical documentation is the canine infection *Dirofilaria immitis* (canine "heart worm"), which has been a major veterinary condition many years. Although experimental models do feature strongly in the history of investigation into filarial infections, these have often been largely directed towards the development of new anti-filarial drugs or immunological aspects rather than on increasing our understanding the pathogenesis and other areas of the pathobiology of these fascinating abundant animals.

The first of the common driving factors, the search for more effective chemotherapeutic regimes, has been catalysed by the fact that the drug effects on the parasites, especially those lying in sensitive tissues, such as those of the skin (where many inflammatory pathways can be activated), often is associated with severe and often life-threatening adverse reactions. Thus, there has been a need to develop safe chemotherapeutic regimes, especially as these treatments are now used in mass drug administration projects where millions of people in OV and LF endemic countries receive these drugs. Understanding these adverse reactions has itself catalysed filarial research and has led to better understanding of the pathogenesis of these infections. One example of this how the acute phases of oncho-dermatitis were clarified—observing the rapid clinical dermal reactions following the administration of the microfilaricidal agent diethylcarbamazine (DEC) enhanced our understanding of the natural responses in the skin when the microfilariae die and cause focal lesions. Likewise, the second of these major driving factors, the attempts to control and eliminate OV and LF, has required a better definition of their epidemiology, and more specifically their rapid detection. In addition, the global elimination programs have catalysed interest in these often ignored chronic diseases in the medical community of endemic countries.

It could be argued that all the interest and support given to endemic country-based elimination programs has ironically been counter-productive to gaining more knowledge on the more fundamental patho-biological aspects of these diseases; pathogenesis and clinical understanding becoming the poor cousins of the major two components, drug development and epidemiological elimination. This is not to say that the advances in these major two components have made has not been in many ways spectacular and a great credit to medicine and allied bodies; they indeed have been, and their major aims are being slowly achieved [3, 4]. There are, however, important facts emerging from various investigation and the sources that are widening our understanding of human filariasis and hopefully this newer information can inform us further as how to more efficiently control, manage and hopefully eliminate the important human filariases.

2. Variations in form and presentation

In attempting to understand filarial infections one is presented with interesting and thought-provoking concepts. Aside from the phenomenon mentioned above of surviving and multiplying usually exclusively within the environment of a preferred host, and often in the vascular system—a preferential location also seen with trematode parasites (e.g., schistosomiasis)—filarial infections can present in different ways, which likely reflects underlying biological differences in host responses, worm stages and other factors. Firstly, there is clear clinical spectrum that ranges from those people who carry increasing parasitic loads with the parasites (microfilariae and adult worms essentially) eventually dying at the end of their life expectancy. This is a situation where there appears to be a developed "tolerance" for these parasites, at least whilst they are alive and generally healthy. This form of the infection, due to the associated focal inflammatory reactions that occur as they eventually die, together with secondary effects (e.g., in OV pruritic irritation and consequent damage from self-scratching), which over a long period of time causes the associated tissues and affected organs to slowly degenerate. In OV this results in the often shown picture of a prematurely aged and atrophic skin, and in LF one sees slow chronic damage to the kidney and other highly vascular structures. At the other end of the clinical spectrum is a highly active condition centred around, at least in OV, very active microfilarial destruction with associated inflammatory events—this is seen in the condition known as "reactive oncho-dermatitis" (ROD) or "sowdah". It has been shown that ROD patients have very strong T-cell based immune responses to *O.volvulus*, whereas those infected people with the steadily increasing parasite load, the degenerative form of the disease, do not have such active T-cell responses. Thus, there is a clinical spectrum that is paralleled in many ways by a corresponding immunological spectrum.

Another variation that exists in filarial infections relates to the host tissue's responses to the different parasitic stages, most being known about the two stages that can be more easily identified in infected people, i.e., the adult forms and microfilarial stage (L1) (**Table 1**). In addition, the host reactions to each of these two stages can be different, and it is probable that changes in the biological status of each of these, or perhaps the host's immunological recognition of these specific stages, are the basis for these differences. Live adult worms appear from histological studies to reside in the tissues with only a minimal cellular response adjacent to at least most for their external surface. Two exceptions occur to this status: firstly, it is very common to find in the tissues associated, although usually not directly in apposition to these adult worms, substantial organised aggregates of lymphoid cells and plasma cells. This indicates in all likelihood that the presence of the adult worm, or at least significant components of this stage, is well recognised by the immune system, although the worm appears to manage to avoid being attacked by host responses through immuno-modulatory mechanisms. Observations in the bovine equivalent of human OV, *Onchocerca gutturosa*, where the female adult worms lie in a serpentine fashion in the epi-ligament membranes lining the nuchal ligament in cattle—the only cellular reactions associated with the live adult worms are again lymphoid cellular aggregates; however, in this case these are located adjacent to the vaginal opening of the female worms suggesting that material emerging from the worms's uterus (which maybe be uterine fluids, microfilariae or microfilarial components) are involved in the induction of this host response. The second major form of observable tissue response to adult worms is that associated with degenerating, or essentially non-viable, adult worms; it should be noted that the definition of nematode viability, and indeed the definition of a live versus a dead filarial worm, is controversial [5]. The cellular responses to degenerating adult filaria is characterised by the typically components of a chronic inflammatory response—e.g., macrophages of different morphologies, and in these cases, eosinophil leucocytes; this is parallel to a classical "foreign body" response in pathological terms. The latter response can be interpreted as resulting from the lack of any immunomodulatory activity being shown by the now inactive adult worm.

The other easily identified parasitic stage, the microfilariae, also is associated with two different tissue reactions: either being alive and free from any cellular reaction, or in contrast degenerating and eliciting very active eosinophil dominant cellular reactions—the latter occurring, for example after the administration of microfilaricidal agents such as DEC and ivermectin. It is thought that when microfilaria emerge from the uterus they change their surface composition which may protect them from host attack [2]. Treatment with microfilaricidal agents probably alters the capability of microfilaria to avoid the host's attack; this is likely the case with the function of ivermectin [6].

Likewise, with LF there is a dramatic range of responses seen clinically, although the mechanisms at play behind this variation are much less clear than those evident in onchocerciasis. There is relatively little data available in humans on the mechanisms behind the variations in those infected individuals that develop clinically obvious lymphoedema or hydrocoele, and those who do not. Suggestions for this difference in clinical presentation have been proposed and these include possible differences on host genetic type, differences in immunological history, and the more general overwhelming of the host's tissues natural ability to recover and absorb the patho-physiological stresses that result from infection and disturbed lymphatic drainage.

3. Changes in our understanding of the pathobiology

The location of filarial worms within the body are thought to be well known and accepted, however it would be judicious to emphasise that our current understanding of this is often based on general assumptions. The adult worms in OV are in general thought to be almost exclusively found in sub-cutaneous tissues, however it should be noted that very few autopsies that have specifically searched for adult worms. The autopsies that have been carried out revealed that adult worms can be found deep in the thigh muscles, in the fascia close to the femoral bone; this location, if it is common, lessens the value of using palpable sub-cutaneous adult containing nodules as an indicator of an individual's paradise load. Another recent finding that questions current thinking has shown that it quite possible that *O.volvulus* migrate and die in lymphatic vessels, those of the dermis, rather than moving in the supporting connective tissue, as was previously presumed [7]. This would support a general concept that virtually all filarial parasites reside in the vascular system. Such a generalisation still needs additional confirmation, especially for filariae such as loiasis, but as histological advances in identifying lymphatic anatomy continues improve this should indeed be possible.

Similarly, with regard the effects of adult LF worms there is a need to adjust long-held understandings. For many years it has been the generally acute concept that adult LF parasites "pack and block" lymphatics inducing lymphoedema. In truth, the complete opposite occurs, with the adult worms stimulating endothelial proliferation and very extensive enlargement of the lymphatic vessels (**Figure 1a** and **b**), rather than physical blockage by these parasites. It is this gross enlargement and expansion of the vessels that leads to their inability to keep the lymph fluid moving forward due to valvular insufficiency; thus, leading to lymph stasis and consequently decreased ability of the dermal tissues to protect the limb and keep it healthy.

The role of host immuno-protective mechanisms in filarial infections is still also not well understood. Histopathological observations in both humans and a rat model provide interesting indications that there is an inflammatory response in the lymphatic walls where the adult worms are residing (**Figure 1a** and **b**) [8]. Experimental studies in rats with secretions from the adult filarial worms showed that the macrophage cellular component of this perivascular host reactions is a likely an important player in the production of factors such as vascular endothelial growth factor (VEGF)—that are known to be elevated in filarial patients—are possibly involved

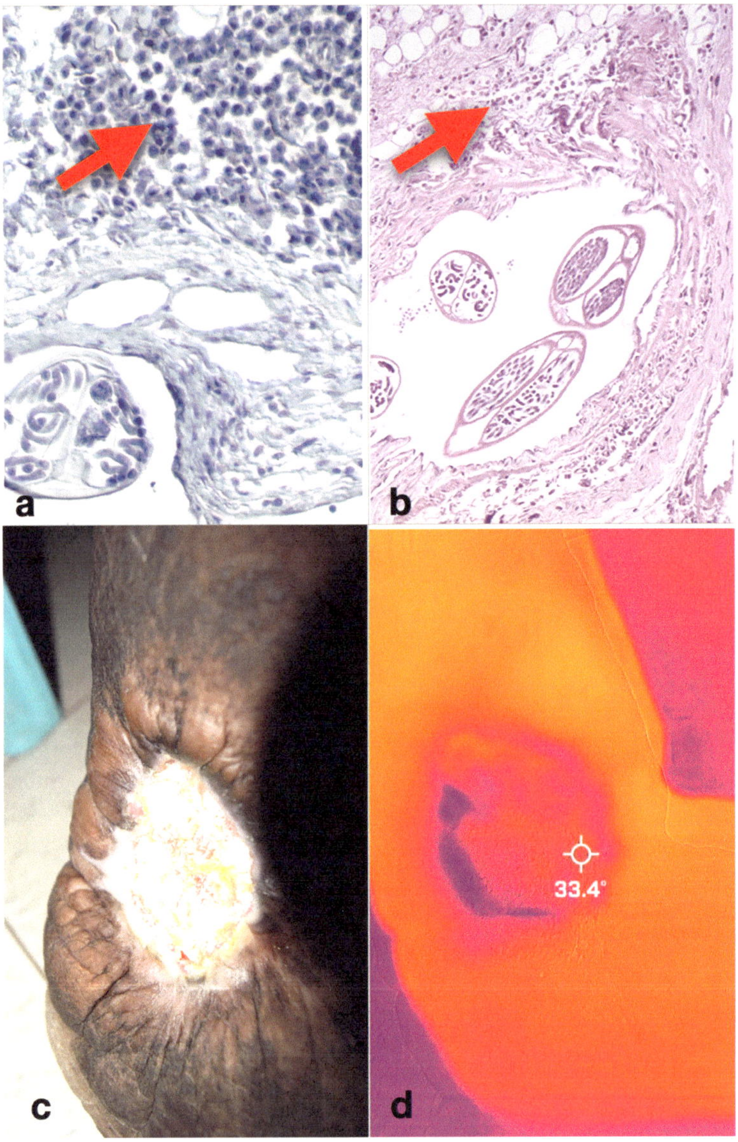

Figure 1.
Filarial infections and consequences; (a) Organised lymphoid aggregates in tissues associated with adult Onchocerca volvulus*; (b) Reactive cells in the walls of the lymphatics carrying Brugia sp. adult worms; (c) Chronic inflamed wound in a lymphoedematous leg; and (d) Thermographic image of the area shown in c. showing temperature differential that shows areas of the wound that are actively inflamed (darker areas).*

in the dramatic lymphatic wall proliferation that is a hallmark of this infection [9]. It is also interesting to note that the tissue reaction that is seen around dead adult *Wuchereria* worms that form "nodules" that often are attached to the internal walls of the affected lymphatics is very similar to that seen around the degenerating adult worms in the sub-dermal nodules of OV. Thus, suggesting the pathological mechanism at play with dead adult worms are similar between parasite species.

There is also support for secondary infections as a major contributor the progression, and perhaps a role in the initial development, of LF. The effectiveness of bacterial and fungal control achieved with the skin hygiene self-care protocol for lymphoedema patients being the major piece of evidence presented to support this contention. It is likely though that the development and progression of lymphoedema has a complex aetiology that includes secondary infections, a parasitic component, certainly in the early stages, and also an important contributor in the marked diminution of the skin and its supporting tissues to be able maintain homeostasis and protect the affected area against external stresses and insults. Understanding the components involved in the pathogenesis of lymphoedema and associated dermal changes would likely greatly enhance the search for much needed new treatments.

Understanding which are the active components of filarial worms that stimulate inflammation, as well as which are the events and mechanisms associated with the prevention of these unwanted reactions, is central to developing better management of these infections. It is likely that microfilaria, and probably other components released from the adult female worm's uterus, stimulate active responses in the host. This may be explanation for the cellular responses seen in tissues adjacent to the uterine opening mentioned earlier. In addition, observations in animal models where the uterus of adult filarial worms have been damaged or blocked, significant cellular reactions do not occur in the tissues where these adult worms reside implying that the uterine components (which include microfilariae, eggshells, etc.) are causes of inflammatory responses. It is important here to mention the role of the common filarial endosymbiont, *Wolbachia*, that is present in at least some filariae (including LF and OV); this organism has been often defined as the major inflammatory component of these parasites. These organisms are indeed an important stimulatory component of these worms but it likely that components other than the endo-symbionts also elicit significant host responses and also contribute to the reactions that occur when these parasites degenerate and release their contents. Another finding that has requires better definition relates to the presence of high levels of circulating immune complexes in at least OV patients [10], and whether these high levels contribute to the immuno-modulation occurring in this disease.

When attempting to understand the host-parasite interactions of an infection it is important to observe the changes and effects as the infections develop in naive individuals (e.g., children and expatriates). Children born and growing up in onchocerciasis endemic areas appear to mount active microfilarial destroying responses that keep the loads of active detectable microfilariae low unit about 7–8 years of age after which the dermal loads begin to significantly increase [1]. This increase likely reflects the mounting ability of the parasite to modulate the host's protective responses against this parasite. Visitors to endemic areas, at least OV endemic areas, who become infected often show acute clinical dermal presentations that reflect reactions to the microfilariae present in their dermal tissues, and these can be quite severe, and these also likely reflect the presence of an active host reaction to the invading parasite.

4. Enhancing program implementation and assessment

An important area that could greatly assist both the OV and the LF programs is to understand the clinical and social effects of these infections, and the current approaches to treatment, have on those individuals affected and on their communities. Monitoring clinical changes over time is a very important approach that has not commonly been carried out. Documenting change in the disease has several valuable outcomes—aside from promoting better individual patient management, showing a reduction in disease has important advocacy implementations for the global elimination program for OV and LF. An additional indicator of success is to monitor the appearance of new cases, where a reduction and an absence reflects the achievement of a successful anthelminthic program.

One of the major challenges to one of the required goals of the GPELF is to provide care to all those suffering from the often devastating two major clinical effects of this infection, i.e., firstly, lymphoedema and dermal pathology (LDP), and secondly hydrocoele (HC) [11]. The WHO has recommended effective protocols for these two conditions—removal of the parasitic cause and a package of skin-focused self-care procedures for lymphoedema and surgical intervention for HC. Registering and training LDP patients, many of whom often live in rural locations that do not have easy access, is challenging. In addition, these patients need to continue their self-care for long periods of time, if not for the remainder of their lives. Hydrocœlectomy surgery, however, is essentially a single event with over 80% success with non-recurrence of the HC, and thus is in managerial terms easier to implement in national programs and is relatively easy to quantitate and report. National programs therefore tend to focus on implementing the surgical component of the morbidity arm of the global efforts against LF rather than lymphoedema care.

As the chemotherapeutic arm of the LF elimination program, i.e., the mass distribution of anthelminthics, is essentially a procedure that should be completed in 5–8 years, and as many LDP patients will need to carry out their self-treatment activities long after the man anthelminthic phase has ended, it has been recommended that LF patient care be integrated in the public health services of endemic countries [11]. This is an appropriate managerial approach but in reality, this is turning out to be difficult to achieve, partially as medical care for a long term, largely chronic, condition that is not immediately life threatening is usually not a high priority for national medical administrations. Thus, a major challenge the national LF Programs must address, in addition to the initial establishment of a LF MMDP program (i.e. Locating LF patients, and making appropriate care available), is to encourage and ensure that LDP patients maintain their self-care over a long-period of time. Understanding how to do this one of the major questions that those wishing to make the global program a complete success need to address: how do we support LDP patients to keep employing the skin care self-care package? Understanding why these patients do not continue their self-care activities, and what support mechanism can be developed to assist their continuance in long-term self-care, are two essential questions that need to be addressed in this goal. Similarly in importance is the development of improved methods to demonstrate any positive clinical effects of these global treatment and elimination efforts on those affected - such as the reduction in the occurrence of new cases, and improvement in existing pathology, would serve well to promote the Program's success.

It is important that modern tests and procedures are developed for assessing filarial patients in routine and special investigations, although it is realised that many, if not most, OV and LF patients reside in areas of the world where medical services are extremely weak if existent at all. Most of the current parameters used for assessment are external in intervention and general in information. It is also likely that approaches that reveal more information about the changes taking place in deeper tissues and organs will be very informative to achieving a better understanding of these infections and their consequences. As mentioned above, it is notable that despite the number of people infected and affected by this infection there are so few documented autopsies available. Ultrasound is commonly used to visualise infected lymphatics and subcutaneous onchocerca nodules, and newer techniques such as optical coherence tomography and Nuclear Magnetic Resonance (NMR) have been used occasionally in investigations in OV or LF.

Externally based parameters are still the most practical of approaches to assess filarial patients in most locations across the endemic zones of the world. It has been found in practice, in our work in Tanzania, that it is important to assess the status of a patient from a holistic point of view, i.e., incorporate together a range of signs, symptoms and appropriate aspects of daily action and mobility. Using a single parameter to assess status or change in status has not been found to be robust enough for carrying out comparisons, either longitudinally in a single patient, or between patients. In OV, there are tools that can be used for both ophthalmologic disease and dermal disease: the presence and change in punctuate keratitis is a useful indicator for the eye, and scoring of the presence and degree of the major dermal changes associated with oncho-dermatitis foe assessing the skin.

With LF induced lymphoedema a common approach is to measure the size/volume of the limb enlargement; this done by either the impractical approach of water displacement, the use of tape measurements of circumferences at standard levels on the limb, or more recently using infra-red [12], or digital volume sensors (such as Lymphotech®) [13]. It should be noted, however, that changes in limb volume can vary considerably over the course of 24 hours, and it is not uncommon for patients who are generally improving to relate that their affected leg "does not weigh as much as it did," although there be no obvious detectable change in affected limb's volume. Incorporating as many quality-of-life parameters (e.g., mobility, duration of working in farms, etc.), are important to use along with the more classical parameters of the observable stage of lymphoedema and dermal change (using the standard described lymphoedema staging scales), and the occurrence of acute filarial attacks (AFA—i.e., increased limb swelling, draining lymph node swelling, feeling "feverish", and other signs and symptoms). It is useful to record not just the occurrence (the number) of acute filarial attacks but also their duration and severity—a reduction in AFA has been found to be a most useful parameter for demonstrating an individual's clinical improvement (**Figure 2**). Another useful tool is thermography to monitor temperature differences in active areas of the dermis [14] (**Figure 1c** and **d**). As this is a condition that stigmatises those it affects, it is important to take steps to address both the stigma the patient feels and any negativeness expressed by the community members where they reside. Active provision of care to those affected in an endemic community affected, and the visibility of seeing patients' improvement, can go a long way to reduce the overall problem of stigma—and secondarily enhance trust in the national program's activities often resulting importantly in higher mass drug administration compliance.

5. Major questions remaining

Understanding the pathobiology of filarial infection is challenging, given their many unique characteristics such as their host specificity and ability to avoid natural defense mechanisms, but this is an intellectually exciting goal, one that is likely to have valuable practical consequences. It is important when addressing this challenge

a. FREQUENCY IN OCCURRENCE OF ACUTE FILARIAL ATTACKS

Reported attacks in the 12 months prior to MDA/Self-care	1.6	0.1 - 2.2
Reported attacks in the period 12-24 months after MDA/Self-care	0.2	0 - 0.3

b.

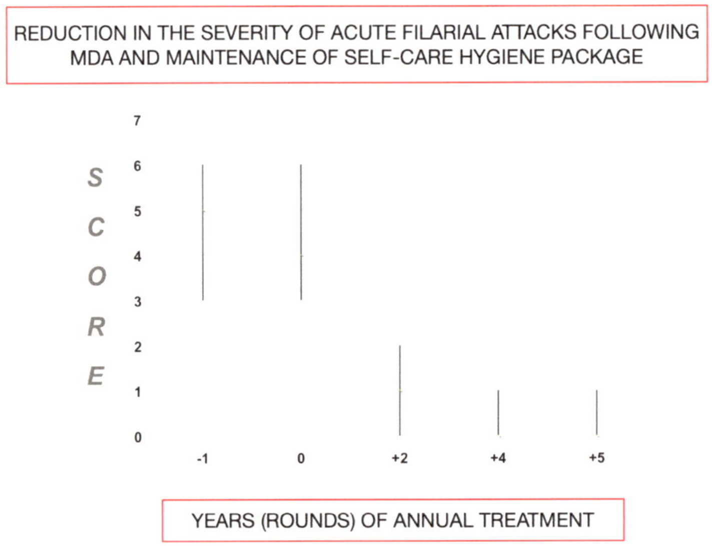

Figure 2.
Acute filarial attacks (a) Change in frequency of filarial attacks in 147 lymphoedema patients after 2 years of receiving the anti-filarial chemotherapy and implementing the recommended self-care hygiene package; and (b) Changes in the clinical presentation of acute filarial attacks in 47 individuals with lymphoedema (47 individuals) following the treatment regime (the assessment score was based on frequency, duration, and severity of the attacks).

to taking a wide approach and to not get over-focussed on specific findings without considering the whole spectrum of the parasite-host interaction, and to keep the major goals in mind—e.g., detection, safe treatment, and reduction in endemicity. A selection of major questions reaming is presented in **Table 2**.

As presented in this discussion it is important to get more data and information about the lesser investigated areas of filarial infections, especially in areas related to understanding the mechanisms in the host-parasite interactions that allow these infections to survive and multiply in sensitive tissues. Currently most of the effort, both politically and fiscally, is being placed on achieving the goal of disease elimination or at least reduction through wide distribution of chemotherapy with some additional supportive approaches (e.g., vector control). A common argument presented is that we do not need to have deeper knowledge of an infection that is being successfully controlled, and now eliminated, from individual countries. In the long-term this may be a valid statement, but we are long way from success extending across the whole OV and LF endemic world, and in addition these drug administration programs are extremely long in duration which is costly. Improved diagnostic tools, more effective means of treating areas

Area of focus	Relevance
What are the differences and commonalities between the different filariae?	Can we make assumptions across filarial sp.?
How do filarial parasites modulate the host's immune system?	Aid in developing better therapies and reduction in parasite loads
Are there unique species specific components that could be used for minimally invasive diagnosis?	Diagnosis and epidemiology
What are the components of filariae that induce inflammatory reactions?	The developing of improved supportive treatments
What are the roles of secondary factors In each filarial disease?	Understanding the complexity if filarial clinical disease
How to best detect the presence of filarial parasites infection in deep tissues?	Improve diagnosis and monitoring of treatment
What is the best practical method to detect and estimate the presence of fertile/actively reproducing filarial parasites?	Central to breaking transmission

Table 2.
Major areas that could be investigated to provide a more detailed information on the patho-biology and detection of the major human filarial infections.

of persistent infection, and more effective treatments (chemotherapeutic agents), could lead to program success much faster than is currently occurring. Addressing any of the questions such as those described in this current discussion would likely contribute positively to improving the activities needed for elimination in many ways (**Table 2**). For example, increasing advocacy for continuing the drug distribution program with donors and recipients by showing clinical improvement in those affected would likely be most advantageous, as would improving the tests used for the detection of cases that are essential for epidemiological assessment that define success.

Although in recent times our understanding of filarial infections has indeed improved, and some fundamental misunderstandings corrected, the emotive classical images of clinical filariases—the grossly swollen limbs, enlarged genitals, and the blind being guided by young children, are unfortunately still often regarded by the public as the current status of these infections. Hopefully this public view will change to one that embraces the success of the recent efforts to understand and reduce this devastating disease. The fact that many LF patients are now receiving treatments that does indeed reduce their morbidity needs to be more generally known. In addition, the observation that in recent years the appearance of new cases of onchocerciasis-induced blindness is now very much frequent needs to be better understood but the public health community.

Acknowledgements

We are indebted to the late Mwele Malecela for her support and most valuable input as a colleague into many of the concepts discussed in this review. Her leadership and scientific knowledge of filarial infections and their treatment was essential to the understandings of filarial disease presented here.

Funding

The publication of this work was supported by the Coalition for Operational Research on Neglected Tropical Diseases (COR-NTD), which is funded at The Task Force for Global Health primarily by the Bill & Melinda Gates Foundation (OPP1190754), by UK aid from the British government, and by the United States Agency for International Development through its Neglected Tropical Diseases Program. Under the grant conditions of the Foundation, a Creative Commons Attribution 4.0 Generic License has already been assigned to the Author Accepted Manuscript version that might arise from this submission.

Author details

Charles D. Mackenzie[1*], Wilfred L. Mandara[2] and Esther Mwakitalu[2]

1 NTD Support Center, Task Force for Global Health, Atlanta, GA, USA

2 National Institute for Medical Research, Ministry of Health, Dar es Salaam, Tanzania

*Address all correspondence to: cmackenzie@taskforce.org

References

[1] Mackenzie CD. Human Filarial Infections: Reflections on the Current Understanding of Their Importance, Pathobiology, and Management. In: Kaminsky R, Geary T, editors. Human and Animal Filariases. Landscape, Challenges, and Approaches for Control. Weinheim, Germany: Wiley-VCH GmbH; 2022. ISBN 9783527346592. Chp.3. 32 pp

[2] Mackenzie CD, Souza A, Geary TG. Diagnosis as assessment of human filarial infections: current status and challenges. In: Kaminsky R, Geary T, editors. Human and Animal Filariases. Landscape, challenges, and approaches for control. Weinheim, Germany: Wiley-VCH GmbH; 2022. ISBN 9783527346592. Chp 5. 21pp

[3] Mackenzie CD, Homeida MM, Hopkins A, Lawrence JC. Elimination of onchocerciasis from Africa: Possible? Trends in Parasitology. 2012;**28**:16-22

[4] Guevara Á, Lovato R, Proaño R, Rodriguez-Perez MA, Unnasch T, Cooper PJ, et al. Elimination of onchocerciasis in Ecuador: Findings of post-treatment surveillance. Parasites & Vectors. 2018;**11**(1):265. DOI: 10.1186/s13071-018-2851-3. PMID: 29690907; PMCID: PMC5937837

[5] Mackenzie CD, Behan-Braman A, Hauptman J, Geary T. Assessing the Viability and Degeneration of the Medically Important Filarial Nematodes. In: Shah MM, Mahamood M, editors. Nematology—Concepts, Diagnosis and Control. 2017. Chp 6: ISBN 978-953-51-3416-9. DOI: 10.5772/intechopen.69512

[6] Moreno Y, Nabhana JF, Solomon J, Mackenzie CD, Geary TG. Ivermectin disrupts the function of the excretory-secretory apparatus in microfilariae of Brugia malayi. Proceedings of the National Academy of Science. 2010;**107**:20120-20125

[7] Mackenzie CD, Huntington MK, Wanji S, Lovato RV, Eversole RR, Geary TG. Association of adult Onchocerca with lymphatic vessels. Journal of Parasitology. 2010;**96**:219-221

[8] Weinkopff T, Mackenzie C, Eversole R, Lammie PJ. Molecular mechanisms of lymphangiectasia in lymphatic filariasis. PLOS Neglected Tropical Diseases. 2014;**8**(7):e2893. DOI: 10.137/ journal. pntd.0002893

[9] Cruickshank JK, Price KM, Mackenzie CD, Spry CJF, Denham DA. Infection of inbred and nude (athymic) rats with Brugia pahangi. Parasite Immunology. 1983;**5**:527-537

[10] Steward MW, Sisley B, Mackenzie CD, El Sheik H. Circulating antigen antibody complexes in onchocerciasis. Clinical & Experimental Immunology. 1982;**48**:17-24

[11] World Health Organisation. Lymphatic Filariasis: Reporting Continued Progress Towards Elimination as A Public Health Problem 2020. Available from: https://www.who.int/news/item/29-10-2020-lymphatic-filariasis-reporting-continued-progress-towards-elimination-as-a-public-health-problem

[12] Zhou C, Yahathugoda C, De Silva L, Rathnapala U, Owen G, Weerasooriya M, et al. Portable infrared imaging for longitudinal limb volume monitoring in patients with lymphatic filariasis. PLoS Neglected Tropical Diseases. 2019;**13**(10):e0007762. DOI: 10.1371/

journal.pntd.0007762. PMID: 31584959; PMCID: PMC6795459

[13] Horton J, Klarmann-Schulz U, Stephens M, Budge PJ, Coulibaly Y, Debrah A, et al. The design and development of a multicentric protocol to investigate the impact of adjunctive doxycycline on the management of peripheral lymphoedema caused by lymphatic filariasis and podoconiosis. Parasites & Vectors. 2020;**13**(1):155. DOI: 10.1186/s13071-020-04024-2. PMID: 32228663; PMCID: PMC7106687

[14] Krishnasastry S, Mackenzie CD. Alternative approaches to lymphoedema care in lymphatic filariasis. PLOS Neglected Tropical Diseases. 2021;**15**(4):e0009293. DOI: 10.1371/journal.pntd.0009293

Chapter 3

Drug Discovery and Development for Soil-Transmitted Helminthiasis: Current Anthelmentics and Compounds in the Pipeline

Eyael Tewelde and Solomon Tadesse

Abstract

Soil-transmitted helminthiasis (STH), one of 20 neglected tropical diseases, afflicts about a quarter of the world's population. A handful of medications, albendazole, mebendazole, pyrantel pamoate, levamisole, and ivermectin, have long constituted the cornerstone of therapy for these infections in both humans and animals. The continuous and long-term reliance on these small range of compounds has led to the emergence of drug resistance in many helminthic strains in animals. The threat of resistance also seems inevitable in humans thereby hampering the World Health Organization's efforts to control or eradicate these neglected tropical illnesses. Hence, there is an urgent need for the discovery and development of new treatment options with broad spectrum activity against various helmintic infections that act *via* novel mechanisms of action. Different strategies are employed in this endeavor which include the identification of promising compounds from natural and synthetic origin, drug repurposing and modification of existing drugs, and vaccine development. The prospect of a "pan-anthelmintic vaccine" also seems encouraging, despite the various obstacles facing the development of vaccines. Here we discuss drug discovery and development efforts for STH.

Keywords: helminthiasis, tropical disease, anthelmintics, parasites, drugs

1. Introduction

Helminthes are large, multicellular, invertebrates with well-developed organ systems with characteristic elongated, flat, or round bodies. This broad range of organisms are mostly active feeders and visible to the naked eye in their adult stages. "Helminth" is a general term for worms. Platyhelminthes (flatworms) and Nemathods (round worms) are recognized as the two parasitologically important phyla (**Figure 1**) of heminths [1–3]. Nematodes, the focus of this book, are unsegmented, long cylindrical worms that are tapered at both ends. The alimentary canal is complete with a mouth

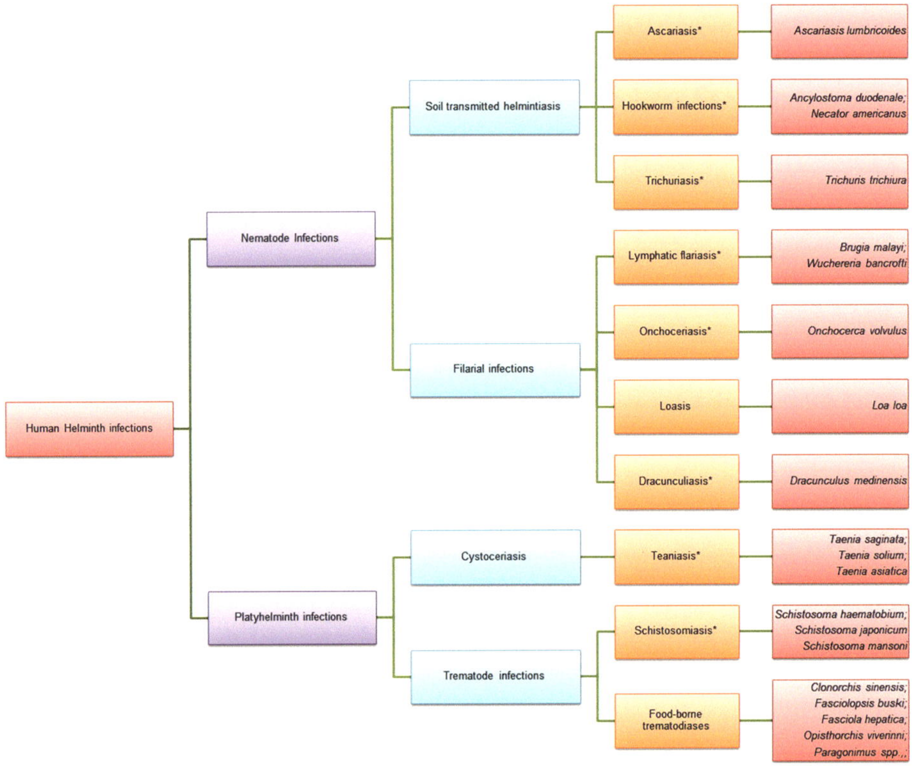

Figure 1.
*Helmintic infections of humans; * Neglected tropical diseases.*

and anus, where a mouth with three lips is present in some intestinal nematodes, and the mouth contains cutting plates in some. Typically, nematodes are bisexual and males are generally smaller. For fertilization, coupling of the sexes is required except for *Strongyloides* [1, 4, 5].

Typically, worms reside in the gastrointestinal tract but may also burrow into other organs like the liver (*Fasciola hepatica*), lung (*Paragonimus westermani*), muscle (*cysticercosis*), skin (*Strongyloides*), lymph (*Wuchereria bancrofti*), eye (*Onchocerca volvulus*), brain (*Paragonimus* sp.), and other tissues [6–8].

Helminths have been affecting human beings throughout the history of mankind and still continue to be major causes of mortality and morbidity [9]. Infections caused by helminthic parasites are among the most widespread infections, affecting a vast population of tropical regions and posing an immense risk to health [10, 11]. In these warm regions, STH are endemic [5].

Ancylostoma duodenale, *Ascaris lumbricoides*, *Necator americanus,* and *Trichuris trichiura* [5], referred to as STH, are the four most important human gastrointestinal nematodes. Infections with STH occur after embryonic eggs or tissues of another host containing larval forms of nematodes are ingested. Eggs passed through feces take about 3 weeks to mature in the soil before they are infectious, hence the name soil-transmitted. Consequently, there is no direct person-to-person transmission, or infection from fresh feces and reinfections occur only as a result of contact with infective stages in the environment [1, 4, 5]. STH is one of the important infections from neglected tropical diseases where 8 out of 20 diseases are caused by helminths [12].

> *Almost 2 billion people (about a quarter of the world's population) are infected with soil-transmitted helminthes worldwide. Approximately 270 million preschool children and more than 550 million school-age children live in areas where these parasites are extensively transmitted. Approximately 250 million girls and adult women are living in areas that are endemic for STH. Infections are widely distributed, with the greatest numbers occurring in sub-Saharan Africa, the Americas and Asia. [5].*

These infections are chronic, mostly asymptomatic, which makes treatment and eradication of the diseases tricky. It can take years for existing infections to resolve, while at the same time, superinfections or reinfections are fairly common occurrences for people who live in endemic communities [13, 14]. According to Wakelin (1996), worms trigger different parasite-mediated immune regulations in the host [2]. Helminthes also evade host immune systems *via* various strategies including motility [15].

In animals, parasitic diseases cause substantial morbidity and mortality worldwide, as well as considerable losses in food production [16]. These diseases are the prime causes of poor livestock productivity in many developing countries [17–19]. In areas where extensive grazing is practiced, helminthic infections are a serious threat to small ruminants resulting in substantial economic losses [20]. Among helminths, nematodes are the most important parasite group of poultry [21], ruminants [16, 19], equids [18, 22, 23], and domestic animals [24].

This chapter discusses the medications in use for STH as well as compounds in the pipeline—preclinical and clinical candidates. Also, it gives insight into the efforts and advances made in the development of vaccines.

2. Treatment of soil-transmitted helminthiasis

Proper hygiene maintenance is one of the most important measures to prevent helminthic infections [25]. At present, the most popular pharmacological means for controlling the disease is the use of anthelmintic drugs [26]. Anthelmintics are drugs that destroy or expel parasitic intestinal worms from the body, by either stunting (vermifuges) or killing (vermicides) [6]. As in all antibiotic drugs, the anthelmintic drugs are expected at metabolic targets that are present in the parasite, but are either absent from or have diverse characteristics than those of the host [4].

Almost all drugs that are used to treat human helminth infections started out as veterinary medication. Antinematoda drugs against pinworm, whipworm, hookworms, ascarids and strongyloides include piperazine, benzimidazoles, imidazothiazoles, tetrahydropyrimidines, macrocyclic lactones, amino-acetonitrile derivatives, spiroindoles, cyclooctadepsipeptides, aminophenylamidines, and organophosphates.

Of the antinematoda medications, the ones used for the treatment of STH are reviewed briefly (**Table 1** and **Figure 2**). Albendazole (**1**), Mebendazole (**2**), Levamisole (**3**), Pyrantel pamoate (**4**), and Ivermectin (**5**) are drugs used in the prevention, treatment, and eradication of STH at different capacities and places. In endemic areas (prevalence >50%), WHO recommends annual/biannual intervention with **1** and **2**. The cure rate for the intervention with benzimidazoles against Ascariasis is high while it is less efficient with Trichiuriasis.

Soil-transmitted helminthiasis	Causative species	Prevalence	DALYs	Treatment option	References
Ascaris	*Ascaris lumbricoides*	820 million	1.33 million	Albendazole Mebendazole Pyrantel pamoate Ivermectin	[5, 27, 28]
Hookworm	*Ancylostoma duodenale* *Necator americanus*	460 million	3.2 million	Albendazole Mebendazole Pyrantel pamoate Levamisole	
Whipworm	*Trichuris trichiura*	440 million	0.65 million	Albendazole Mebendazole Ivermectin	

Table 1.
Epidemiology and treatment options of soil-transmitted helmintiasis.

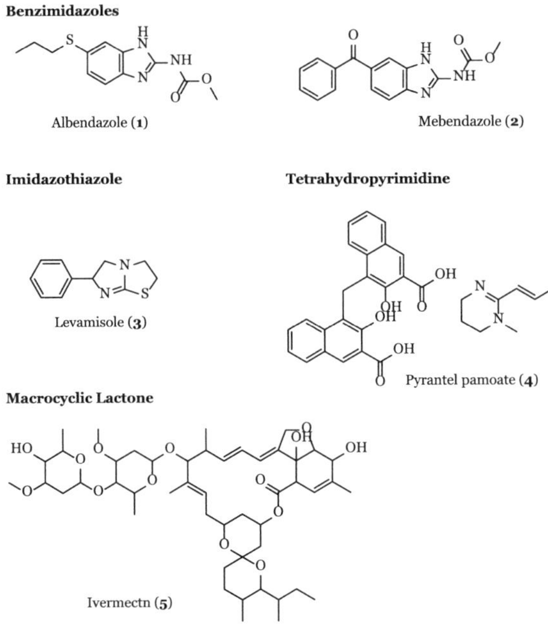

Figure 2.
Chemical structures of anthelmintics used for STH treatment.

2.1 Benzimidazoles

Benzimidazoles are Benzo derivatives of Immidazole. The name benzimidazole is the most popular yet the terms benziminazole, benzoglyoxaline, and 1,3-benzdiazole are also used to describe the compound class. This pharmacophore is found in lots of bioactive compounds with different biological activities. Since the mid-1990s, the therapeutic potential of the class has been and continues to be explored. A range of compounds are approved and available for varied clinical uses with this heterocyclic nucleus. The different derivatives with their varied uses (antimicrobial, antiparasitic, antihypertensive, anti-inflammatory, anticancer, and antiulcer) and their modes of action are compiled and available in a number of publications [29–32].

One of the benzimidazoles approved clinical uses is as anthelmintic drugs. They are the only true broad-spectrum antibiotics active against nematodes, trematodes, and to some extent cestodes. The discovery of thiabendazole in 1961 [33] and its approval as anthelmintic revolutionized treatment. In the years that followed, hundreds of benzimidazoles were synthesized but only a few evolved to be drugs.

Shortly after its discovery, it was found that thiabendazole undergoes enzymatic hydroxylation which renders it inactive [34]. To overcome this problem, investigators began to prepare second-generation benzimidazoles with structural modifications that might prevent metabolic inactivation. Combinations of the modifications at positions 2- and 5- of the molecule have provided the most active drugs [35]. Albendazole (**1**) and mebendazole (**2**) are among the successful compounds of the class.

The mode of action of these drugs is inhibition of microtubule polymerization [36, 37]. This is believed to be a result of the pseudo irreversible binding of the monomer tubulin which prohibits aggregation. This results in the observed effects, including inhibition of cellular transport and energy metabolism. Inhibition of these secondary events appears to play an essential role in the lethal effect on worms. Benzimidazoles progressively deplete energy reserves and inhibit the excretion of waste products and protective factors from parasite cells.

As these changes coincided with the disappearance of cytoplasmic microtubules, it was suggested that benzimidazoles act by inhibiting the microtubule-mediated transport of secretory vesicles in the helminth absorptive tissues with the released digestive enzymes being responsible for the observed tissue damage. The safety of these drugs is astounding considering tubulin is a ubiquitous protein. The principle of the high selective toxicity of benzimidazole anthelmintics is not entirely clear but it appears primarily to be due to the much stronger and irreversible binding interaction of the drugs with helminth as compared with mammalian tubulins [36]. Unfortunately, animal parasites with mutations in the β-tubulin gene have become resistant to benzimidazoles and other anthelmintics.

2.2 Imidazothiazole

The imidazothiazole nucleus is active against a broad range of nematodes yet does not have any efficacy toward flukes or tapeworms. The first of this class is the racemic mixture tetramisole. Later, it was found that the L-isomer, Levamisole (**3**), was much more active than both the racemic mixture and the D-isomer. To date, it is the only one of the classes to be used for clinical use [38].

The imidazothiazoles are nicotinic anthelmintics that act as agonists at nicotinic acetylcholine receptors (nACHR) of nematodes. Their anthelmintic activity is mainly attributed to their ganglion-stimulant (cholinomimetic) activity, whereby they stimulate ganglion-like structures in somatic muscle cells of nematodes. This stimulation first results in sustained muscle contractions, followed by a neuromuscular depolarizing blockade resulting in paralysis. The spastic paralysis of the worm results in its expulsion from the host. The detailed mode of action for **3** was investigated using the patch-clamp technique that at the single-channel level in *Ascaris suum* muscles, it causes activation of cation-selective channels, in addition to voltage-sensitive open channel-block and desensitization [39–41].

After the discovery, **3** has seen success over the years as an anthelmintic treatment both for veterinary and human use. The compound also has an immunomodulatory effect and has been approved as adjuvant therapy for cancer treatment [38]. Despite the compound's efficacy for various conditions, it has a variety of side effects. The US FDA has dropped the drug from the market in the USA because of the side effects, yet it continues to be a treatment option in many countries as an anthelmintic.

2.3 Tetrahydropyrimidines

The first compound of this class, pyrantel (**4**), was introduced in 1966 as an anthelmintic. It however did not possess activity against whipworm [42]. To tackle this lack of efficacy derivatives of the compound were synthesized [43].

This group of antinematoda drugs shares the mode of action of imidazothiazoles. They are nicotinic agonists [44] possibly at the same receptor. Compounds of this class including **4**, like **3** activate the L-subtype nAChRs in *A. suum* while some preferentially activate the N-subtype. Because of their levamisole-type pharmacological action, these groups of compounds also share the toxicity of imidazothiazoles.

2.4 Macrocyclic lactones

Avermectins and milbemycins (which are deglycosylated analogs) are the anthelmintic macrocyclic lactones. The avermectins and milbemycins are the macrolides produced through fermentation by soil-dwelling microorganism *Streptomyces avermitilis* [39]. MLs were introduced in the 1980s as antiparasitic agents with broad spectrum activity against nematodes and arthropods. It is a unique combination of killing both endo and ectoparasites affording them the name "edectocides" [44, 45]. Ivermectin (**5**), the semisynthetic derivative of abamectin, is one of the commercially available avermectin and the first and only approved endectocide for human use.

The macrocyclic lactones induce a reduction in motor activity and paralysis in both arthropods and nematodes. The parasitic effects are mediated through GABA and/or glutamate-gated chloride channels (GluCl), collectively known as ligand-gated chloride channels [46]. The endectocides cause paralysis and death of both arthropod and nematode parasites due to their paralytic effects on the pharyngeal pump which affects nutrient ingestion, and on the parasite somatic musculature limiting its ability to remain at the site of predilection in the host. In addition, MLs cause inhibitory effects on the female reproductive system and cause reductions in parasite egg production [40, 41, 47, 48].

3. Need for new medication

Anthelmintic pharmacologic treatment options are few. Albeit very successful until recently, the chemicals used in the group of diseases are limited in number. The continuous and long-term reliance on these small range of compounds has led to the development of drug resistance in many helminthic strains [11, 18, 48, 49]. Resistance is observed in all classes of antinematoda drugs in animals.

Though resistance to STH and other nematode infections in humans has not been reported, reduced efficacy and low cure rates are observed in some endemic parts of the world. Cross-resistance, which is helminths developing resistance to two or more drugs with similar modes of action without direct previous exposure and side-resistance, where resistance develops for the same chemical family although belonging to different chemical groups, are common occurrences [50]. Hence, "resistance is inevitable" and better detection of the emergence of resistant helminths and devised strategies to cope with them once they do appear, should be in place [51].

Additionally, for a certain set of patients, such as pregnant and lactating mothers, certain anthelmintic medicines are contraindicated. These medications should also be used with caution in patients with hepatitis and in children under 2 years of age [11]. Although safety profiles for anthelmintic drugs are compelling, there still remains a lot unknown about their teratogenicity and embryotoxicity. Hence, there is no drug approved for treatment or prevention in the first trimester of pregnancy. There also exists ambiguity in the ethics of exposing women of reproductive age to such drugs [52]. To combat the above-stated challenges in anthelmintic treatment, the availability of new anthelmintic therapy will be essential over the next few years.

4. Drug discovery and compounds in the pipeline

Development of more effective medicines and medicine to improve patient outcomes and in case of drug resistance of STH is stated as one of three critical actions in the roadmap to ending the neglect to attain the sustainable development goals [12]. Therefore, considerable efforts have been devoted to the development of new anthelmintic drugs, especially those with more pronounced efficacy in nematodes resistant to classical anthelmintics. The efforts, routes explored, promising results, challenges, and opportunities along the path of anthelmintic drug discovery are discussed in reviews [53, 54]. Drug discovery and approval of anthelmintic medication that can be used for human use have lagged behind for the past two decades except for the approval of two compounds (**Figure 3**).

Various approaches are used to this end. The synthetic approach has been the most successful in the past in particular with anthelmintic compounds. It is still continues to be one of the mainstays of drug discovery. The other route is finding effective treatment options from natural remedies and compounds from natural products. Drug repurposing from veterinary anthelmintics and medications for other indications, and combinations of existing anthelmintic medication are the other endeavors affording the promise of better control.

4.1 Natural products

Nature is a farm of unique compounds. A number of inimitable bioactive molecules have been isolated from natural sources. In the past few decades, however, natural product drug discovery has taken a backseat. According to Jayawardene et al.

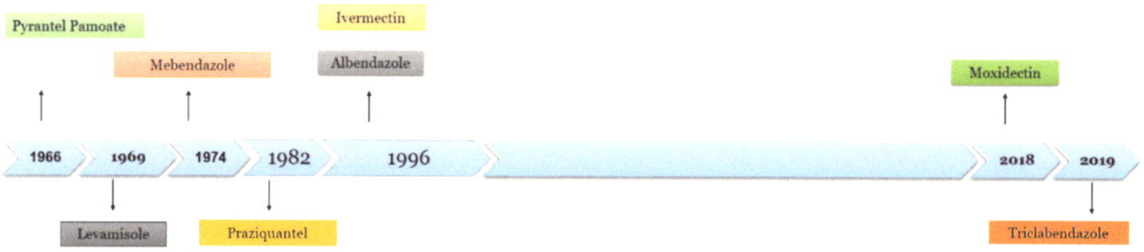

Figure 3.
Timeline of approval of anthelmintics used for nematode infections in human.

difficulties in access and supply, complexities of natural product chemistry, concerns about intellectual property rights, and greater optimism of success with collections of compounds prepared by combinatorial chemistry methods are the main reasons [55].

Recently, the interest in natural products as drug leads is being revitalized since technological and scientific developments are addressing some of the challenges [56]. In terms of anthelmintic drug discovery, the discovery and success of ivermectin hugely impacted the research in favor of natural products [57]. Over the past two decades, a vast number of plant species have been tested against parasitic nematodes such as *Haemonchus contortus*, *A. suum*, *A. lumbricoides*, and non-parasitic free-living nematodes like *Caenorhabditis elegans* and *Pheretima posthuman* [55]. Compounds from natural compounds with promising antinematoda activity (**Figure 4**) are discussed.

Screening of 7500 plant extracts from a library resulted in four αpyrones from two active plant extracts. Goniothalamin (**6**) from *Cryptocarya novoguineensis* and three kavalactones from *Piper methysticum* namely dihydrokavain (**7**), desmethoxyyangonin (**8**), and yangonin (**9**), were purified. All four compounds affected *H. contortus* in an irreversible manner at different stages of the nematode [58]. In a follow-up study, the latter two kavalactones were synthesized with 17 analogs to study the structure–activity relationships. Four of synthesized analogs showed activities far greater than either of the parent compounds. All the synthesized compounds including the original kavalactones did not show toxicity against human HepG2 hepatoma cells *in vitro* with the most potent derivative showing the most selectivity [59].

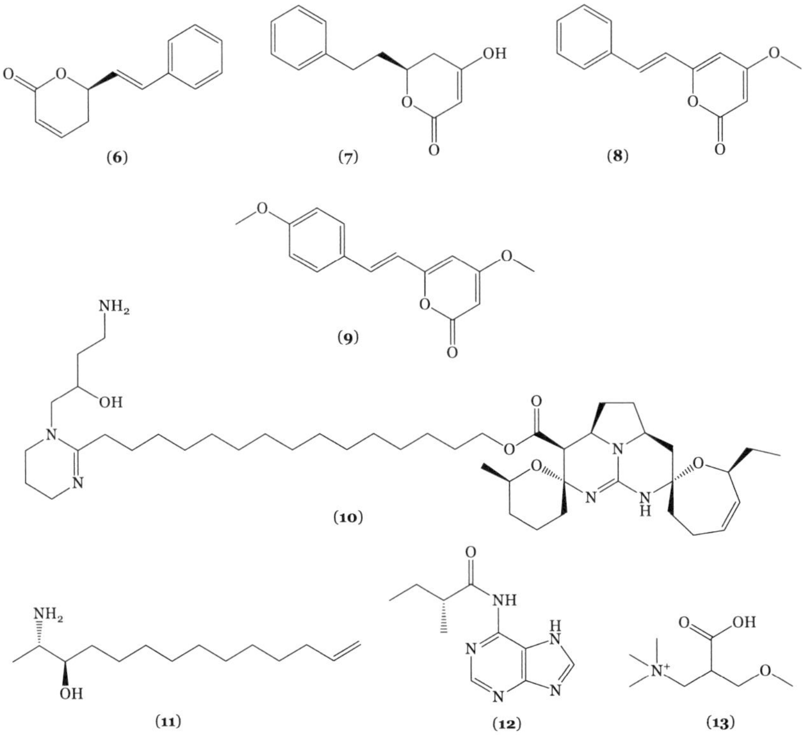

Figure 4.
Natural compounds with anthelmintic activity.

A diverse set of natural compounds with prodigious potential to drug discovery is marine compounds. Fromiamycalin (**10**) from *Monanchora unguiculata*, halaminol A (**11**) from *Haliclona* sp. [60], phorioadenine A (**12**) from *Phoriospongia* sp. [61], and echinobetaine B (**13**) from *Echinodictyum* sp. [62] are anthelmintic compounds from marine sponges. The preliminary SAR of the two latter nematicides revealed the importance of the N-acyl side chain in compound **12** and the importance of 2-OMe and stereopurity of the pharmacophore.

4.2 Synthetic compounds

The synthesis of new compounds is a fruitful undertaking in terms of discovering new therapeutic options with novel mode of action [63]. Promising compounds from this undertaking are discussed (**Figure 5**). High throughput screenings of synthetic compounds and libraries have afforded a number of actives. Though this process of drug development is lengthy and expensive, it is still one of the most rewarding strategies.

Screening of molecules from compound libraries has afforded "Hit" compounds for further development and optimization. Discussed below are the promising compounds under development from this venture. Screening of 67,012 compounds in one non-parasitic, two parasitic nematode species, and two vertebrate models (HEK293 cells and zebrafish), identified 30 structurally distinct anthelmintic lead molecules. The family labeled Wact-11 was found to inhibit complex II at the Q-site with nematode specificity and nanomolar potency [64].

The ChemBridge DIVERset and Maybridge Hitfinder compound libraries of 26,000 compounds were screened affording 14 compounds anthelmintic actives with

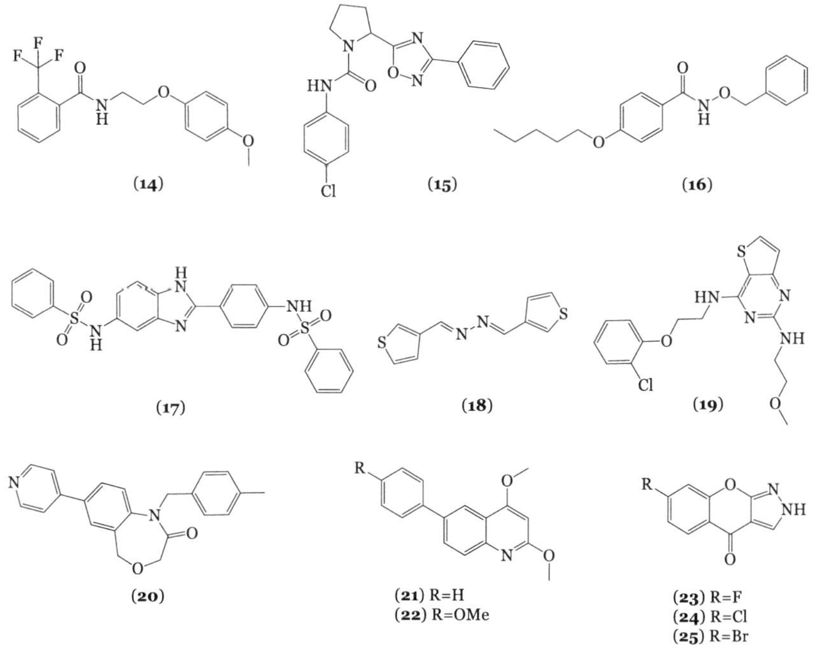

Figure 5.
Synthetic compounds with anthelmintic activity.

5 of them having high nematode specificity [63]. Of the nematode selective compounds, CID 2747322 (**14**) was shown to act in a different biochemical pathway than benzimidazole, levamisole, ivermectin, and amino-acetonitrile derivatives. Following this, a structure–activity relationship study established the complex II inhibition action of the compound class, benzamide analogs [65, 66]. The study highlighted the relevance of the amide group for nematicide activity [66].

The "Open Scaffolds" library was screened for anthelmintic activity and the compound 1-methyl-1H-pyrazole-5-carboxamide, called SN00797439 (**15**), was identified as a "hit" compound exhibiting broad range activity [67]. Following this discovery, structural optimization of the hit compound SN00797439, resulted in the discovery of a pyrrolidine-oxadiazole series with the potential to become a novel class of anthelmintics because their potency is already on the level of commercial anthelmintics, with a significant cytotoxicity window and evidence that a broad anthelmintic spectrum is achievable. Current efforts are directed toward progressing the best compounds and assessing their efficacy and toxicity *in vivo* [68–70].

Screening of the "Kruz box," 236 compounds from diverse chemical classes, afforded two compounds designated BLK127 (**16**) and HBK4 (**17**) that induced phenotypic changes in infective larval stages of *H. contortus*. Interestingly, compound BLK127 exerted a phenotype that was similar to a recently described lethal evisceration phenotype. HBK4, a benzimidaxole derivative, was markedly more potent on L4s than L3s [71]. In a consequent study, BLK127 was found to decrease the viability of adult *H. contortus* both in sensitive and resistant strains and showed no hepatotoxic effect, even at the highest concentration tested while HBK4 had no impact on the viability of adults and exhibited significant hepatotoxicity. The benzyloxy amide was more extensively metabolized with a glycine conjugate of 4-(pentyloxy)benzoic acid as the main BLK127 metabolite in ovine liver yet the biotransformation was found to be low in both strains of the nematode with no significant difference [63].

Five compounds, with scaffolds not described as nematicidal prior, were found to be active against *C. elegans* in testing a library of 175 compounds. One of the five actives, (1E,2E)-1,2-bis(thiophen-3-ylmethylene)hydrazine (**18**), was active as a nematicide, but innocuous to the vertebrate model zebrafish. Conjugation of an unsaturation (one or two double bonds) with an electronegative atom in the center of the molecule (N, O, or S) and an aromatic ring were observed patterns in 26 of 28 active compounds indicating that this type of structure constitutes a scaffold for future optimization. It is also important to highlight that five out of the six most potent nematicides were symmetric, with five-atom aromatic heterocycles as substituents [72].

Screening of 480 small-molecule compound libraries (Chemistry Research Laboratory, University of Oxford) against both eggs and adults of *Trichuris* parasites revealed two active chemotypes, one with a diaminothienopyrimidine scaffold [73]. OX02926 (**19**), 2,4-diaminothieno[3,2-d] pyrimidine, and three close neighbors exhibited activity. Though the compound reaches the activity threshold for lead compounds for drug development against the microfilarial nematode its small selectivity window of their activity against the parasite compared to cytotoxicity in a mammalian cell line needs particular attention. Other thienopyrimidines have broad utility in medicinal chemistry, but have not previously been described as having an anthelmintic activity which could mitigate the cost of drug development [73].

The other chemotype with the dihydrobenzoxazepinone scaffold, OX02983 (**20**), was effective at reducing the ability of eggs to establish infection *in vivo*, thus pointing the way to a potential environmental treatment for trichuriasis [74]. In efforts of improving efficacy, dihydrobenzoxazepinones analogs of OX02983 were studied affording an understanding of the SAR of the chemical group. From the study dihydrobenzoquinolinones are suggested as possible candidates for further improvement. It was demonstrated that the class of compounds and related compounds were active against multiple helminths across different phyla: nematodes and trematodes. The improvement of potency is still a point of progress [75].

Two 6-arylquinolines (**21** and **22**) showed activity comparable in potency to the nematicide levamisole against susceptible strains of *H. contortus*. These compounds were also active against the various drug-resistant strains. Evidence of activity against the important parasitic nematodes *T. colubriformis* and *O. circumcincta* was also reported [76]. 7-fluoro-(**23**), 7-chloro-(**24**), 7-bromo-(**25**) derivatives of benzopyrano[2,3-c]pyrazol-4(2H)-one also showed potent anthelmintic activities against the model nematode *C. elegans*. Although the compounds were not -cidal they strongly inhibited the development of nematodes, with the majority of larvae never progressing past the L1 stage. They also showed favorable toxicity toward the worms than human cell lines [77].

4.3 Drug repurposing and modification of existing drugs

Drug repurposing (also called drug repositioning, drug re-profiling, drug re-tasking, and therapeutic switching) is the process of developing new indications for existing drugs to achieve optimal potential and maximize the value of a therapeutic drug. Repositioned drugs include marketed drugs that are still under patent or patents that have expired, drugs that have moved through development and fallen at clinical or regulatory hurdles, and stereoisomers or metabolites of existing compounds. Drug repurposing accelerates the drug discovery and development process with relatively lower costs and reduced risks of failure since the molecules have existing clinical and/or preclinical data [78, 79]. Though the strategy is expected to let the most use out of the already known compounds a lot of hurdles like resources and access to information keep us from reaping the full benefits; the challenges and opportunities toward this undertaking are reported in Pushpakom et al.

In anthelmintic drug repurposing the main effort is to prove the efficacy of known anthelmintics for other helminth species in hopes of broader spectrum activity and cross-over development of veterinary anthelmintics for human use (**Figure 6**) [80]. A review by panic et al. reported the ongoing efforts for the approval of the benzimidazoles (flubendazole (**26**), fenbendazole (**27**), oxibendazole (**28**)), emodepsin (**29**), oxantel pamoate (**30**), tribendimidine (**31**), doramectin (**32**), and melbemycin (**33**) for human STH. The review also gives insight to the repositioning efforts of nitrazoxanide (**34**) and cyclosporine (**35**).

Emodepsin, the antnematoda cyclodepsipeptide approved for use in cats, has been shown to be effective in human models for STH. In nematodes, the over-activation of the SLO-1 receptors by **29** is likely to induce a potassium efflux triggering a hyperpolarization of the neurons that results in a decreased synaptic transmission and muscle contraction, leading notably to a paralysis of the worm pharynx [81]. The drug is currently in clinical trials for *T. trichiura* and Hookworm infections in adults (ClinicalTrials.gov).

Furthermore, **29** and its precursor, PF1022A (**36**), were found to be fully effective against benzimidazole-, levamisole- and ivermectin-resistant populations of *H. contortus* in sheep as well as an ivermectin-resistant *C. oncophora* population in cattle

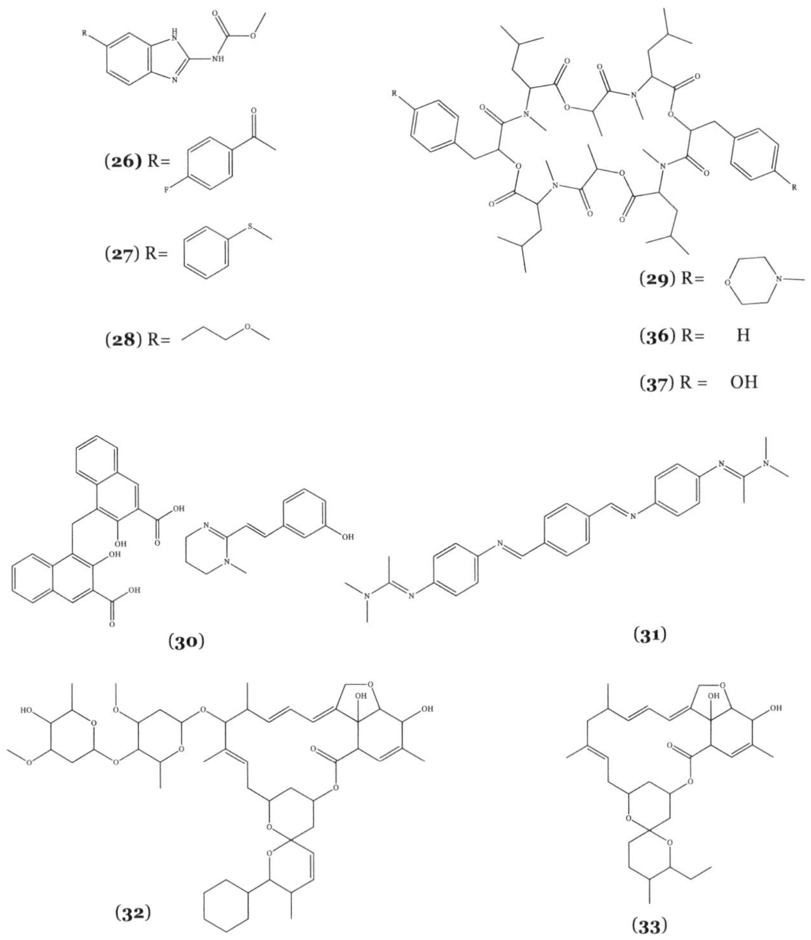

Figure 6.
Veterinary anthelmintics investigated for repurposing to human anthelmintics.

which reinforces endeavor [82]. Compound **36**, isolated from cultured mycelia of *Mycelia sterilia* is described to have a different mode of action from the known anthelmintics which makes it ideal for the development of new medication [83, 84]. The compound is also shown to be effective in human STH models [85]. PF1022H (**37**) is a bis-hydroxy derivative of **36**, which perhaps represents an interesting precursor for new related anthelmintics [86].

In the effort for repurposing other compounds active for various other conditions are investigated for their anthelmintic activities and proved effective (**Figure 7**). Sertraline (**38**), paroxetine (**39**), and chlorpromazine (**40**), are antidepressant and antipsychotic medications that exhibited anthelmintic activity across a broad range of nematode (both free-living and parasitic) and trematode species. The drugs were active on nematodes resistant to existing anthelmintics that target ion channels and microtubules. Furthermore, mutations in the genes responsible for these drugs' anti-depressant or anti-psychotic effects in humans did not eliminate their anthelmintic actions. The findings suggest the modes of anthelmintic action of the compounds might perhaps be novel, which warrants further investigation [87].

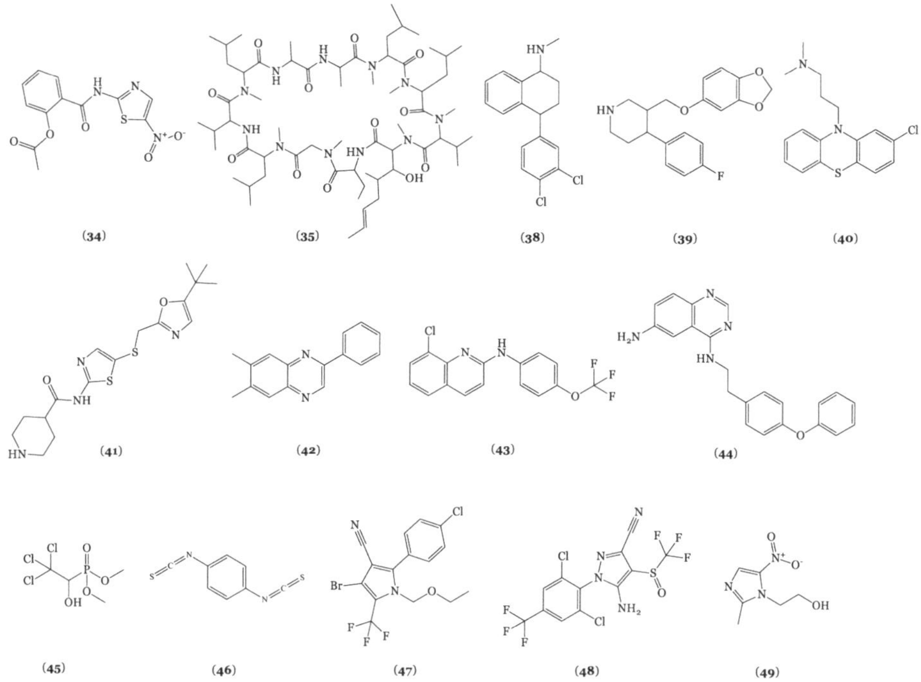

Figure 7.
Drugs and compounds of other indications investigated for repurposing to anthelmintics.

SNS-032 (**41**) and AG-1295 (**42**) are kinase inhibitors identified for their anthelmintic activities against *H. contortus* while screening the "stasis box." Compound **41** is cyclin-dependent kinase (CDK)-2, −7, and -9 inhibitor and entered phase I clinical trials. Compound **42**, a 6,7-dimethyl-2-phenylquinoxaline, is a protein tyrosine kinase (PTK) inhibitor targeting the platelet-derived growth factor (PDGF) receptor kinase. Both compounds showed comparable activities but the former has a higher toxicity profile [88]. Hence, SAR study of tetrahydroquinoxaline chemical series, **42** and its 14 analogs, was attempted. All compounds were shown to have inhibitory effects on larval motility, development, and growth, and induced evisceration through the excretory pore in xL3s. Though the typical kinase (PTK) was not characterized in the test nematode the results point to a mode of action involving dysregulation of morphogenetic processes during a critical time frame, in agreement with the expected behavior of a tyrosine kinase inhibitor [89]. Currently, the metabolism, resistance level, and mechanism of action of these candidates are being tested.

A quinoline derivative, ABX464 (**43**), was found to be active aganist *H. contortus* and *C. elegans* from the "pandemic response box." The potent *in vitro* effect on the most pathogenic and reproductively active stage of *H. contortus* encourages the optimization of **43** *via* SAR studies and toxicity evaluation of analogs with increased potency. The compound was first reported as a novel anti-HIV molecule [90] and is now undergoing phase 2 clinical trials as an anti-inflammatory compound for the treatment of ulcerative colitis, Crohn's disease, and rheumatoid arthritis in humans (ClinicalTrials.gov, NIH). Currently, the mechanism of action of the compound in nematodes is unknown, but could be explored using genomic, transcriptomic, and/or proteomic methods [91].

EVP4593 (**44**) was found to be a promising hit of four hits out of a library 2745 compounds discovered from a repurposing library owing to its potent anthelmintic activity and favorable cytotoxicity. Though no *in vivo* studies have been reported, considering its novel and unexplored chemical scaffold for anthelmintic activity, the observed broad anthelmintic profile, and its relatively high selectivity index, the compound may be an interesting starting point for further optimization [92].

Screening of 1600 FDA-approved compounds revealed two active compounds, trichlorfon (**45**) and bitoscanate (**46**), against hookworm and *Trichurus* species *in vivo*. Though the compounds have clear limitations, related pharmacophores could be of value [93]. Thirty-two hit molecules, of which 30 were analogs of the commercial product chlorfenapyr (**47**), were identified from a library of pesticide analogs. The mode of anthelmintic action is expressed to be similar to the compound class's insecticidal action which is oxidative phosphorylation. The other two potent inhibitors of *H. contortus* motility were derivatives of fipronil (**48**). The latter two had higher cytotoxicity while the arylpyrrole derivatives showed less cytotoxicity [94].

Metronidazole (**49**) and derivatives exhibited anthelmintic activity comparable with that of albendazole and can be further developed as alternative anthelmintic agents to combat drug resistance that will certainly follow the use of monotherapy in treating helminthiasis [95].

Another approach for drug discovery is the modification of already existing anthelmintic drugs (**Figure 8**) to improve their efficacy and/or bioavailablity. 1,2,5-tri-substituted benzimidazole derivatives (**50**), affected adult worm motility more than albendazole. Because of substitution in these compounds would not meet the structure–activity relationships conditions necessary to bind to tubulins at the anthelmintic benzimidazole binding site. These new benzimidazole derivatives could bind tubulins at a different site from 2-methyl-benzimidazole carbamate, or present a different drug target, so further studies should be conducted to identify the pharmacological target of these potential anthelmintic compounds [96]. Another modification on the benzimidazole scaffold, a coumarin-benzimidazole hybrid (**51**), was found to paralyze earthworms equipotent to albendazole. Also, its mortality activity was marginally greater than the activity of albendazole at all concentrations. The activity was in agreement with prediction of activity spectrum of substances (PASS) projections. In addition, a comparative analysis of calculated Lipinski's parameters reveals that the compound has the propensity to be orally bioavailable [97]. Similarly, organometallic derivatives of albendazole were synthesized and tested for their anthelmintic activities. *T. muris* and *H. conturtus* were the two nematodes in the collection of parasites. Two compounds showed some activity toward the former but none of the analogs were active against the latter [98].

Tenvermectin (**52**) is a macrolide designed after successful avermectins. It was obtained from a genetically engineered *S. avermitilis* [99]. The components tenvermectin A and B were found to be effective in expelling *Ascaris* and *Trichuris* sp. with tenvermectin A being less toxic than ivermectin [100].

4.4 Combination of existing anthelmintics

Combination of anthelmintics is another approach being investigated to increase the effectiveness of therapies and avoid or delay resistance. Drugs of different classes with different modes of action are combined to achieve better eradication of nematodes. Combination of moxidectin and albendazole for Trichuriasis is in clinical trials (ClinicalTrials.gov). Another combination investigated is oxantel pamoate

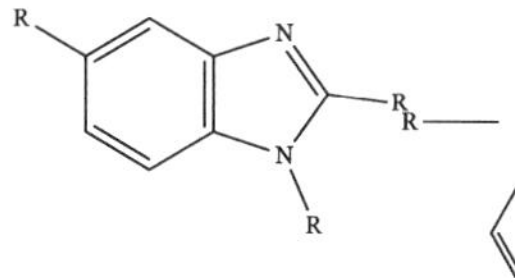

(50)

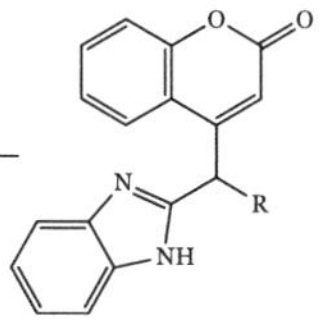

(51)

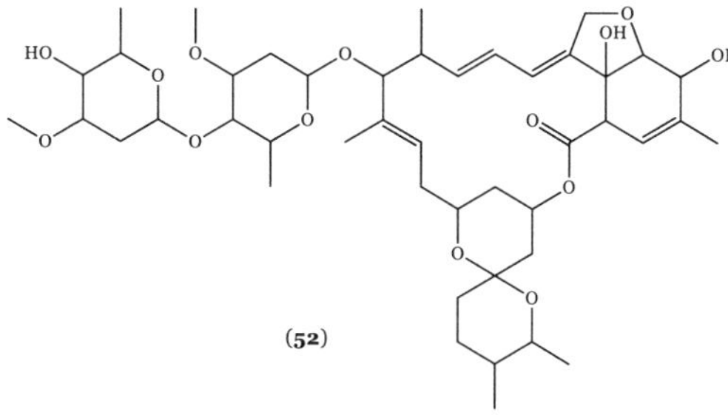

(52)

Figure 8.
Modification of already existing anthelmintic drugs for new anthelmintic discovery.

with albendazole, mebendazole, and ivermectin for the treatment of tricuriasis and hookworm infections [101]. Triple therapy with albendazole, pyrantel pamoate, and oxantel pamoate is also stated to be more efficacious and tolerable in *T. trichuria* infections [102]. Combination therapies are considered in the condition that there does not exist resistance of all members of the combination.

5. Vaccine development

As the global community strives to meet the target set for neglected tropical diseases in 2030, different strategies are set [12]. In parallel with environmental sanitation and hygiene intervention, mass deworming campaigns are undertaken in endemic areas. Despite making significant progress in reducing the burden of STH, deworming campaigns raise concerns about their long-term viability and the emergence of resistance. In addition, medications available at present fail to offer long-term protection against reinfection [15, 27]. Vaccination presents an attractive alternative for controlling STH infections because it allows for the interruption of infection, disease, and transmission in a single step [27]. The development of anthelmintic vaccines is fraud with hurdles. Selecting lead antigens, selection of adjuvants, mass production, efficacy, immunogenicity, and safety are some of the difficulties. The progress, challenges, lessons learned, and future perspectives of STH-vaccine development are reviewed in multiple articles [15, 103, 104].

Anthelmintic lead selections are more complex compared to vaccines for other anti-infectives because of the multiple life cycle stages of helminths each with stage specific antigen. As reviewed by Zawawi and Else, there are four types of anthelmintic leads [103]. Crude antigen preparations, irradiated extracellular vesicles/secretions, are native parasite molecules which sit at the host–parasite interface that induce immune responses. Recombinant proteins and DNA-based preparations are the other two lead antigens in the works. These are expressed to be safer and more convenient than crude preparations. Two recombinant protein vaccine candidates, Na-APR-1 and Na-GST, against the hookworm *N. americanus* are currently in clinical trials (ClinicalTrials.gov) for human use.

Epitopes are the fourth lead antigen molecule. They are identified via reversed volcanology approach based on immunological and bioinformatics tools. Antigens identified *via* these technologies are found to be stage specific and essential for the parasite biological process. MHC-II T-cell epitopes from *T. trichiura* genome sequence were identified *in silico*, incorporated into virus-like particles and tested *in vivo* in murine models. Vaccination results confirm epitope-based vaccines to be promising for development [105]. Another highly anticipated endeavor is the "pan-anthelmintic vaccine" which is to contain a combination of antigen or a consensus of antigens against all four STH as co-infections with two or more of the species is a common occurrence in endemic areas [106].

Author details

Eyael Tewelde and Solomon Tadesse*
Department of Pharmaceutical Chemistry and Pharmacognosy, School of Pharmacy, College of Health Sciences, Addis Ababa University, Addis Ababa, Ethiopia

*Address all correspondence to: solomon.tadesse@aau.edu.et

References

[1] Castro GA. Helminths: Structure, classification, growth, and development. In: Baron S, editor. Medical Microbiology. 4th ed. Galveston (TX): University of Texas Medical Branch at Galveston; 1996. Chapter 86. Available from: https://www.ncbi.nlm.nih.gov/books/NBK8282/

[2] Wakelin D. Helminths: Pathogenesis and defenses. In: Baron S, editor. Medical Microbiology. 4th ed. Galveston (TX): University of Texas Medical Branch at Galveston; 1996. Chapter 87. Available from: https://www.ncbi.nlm.nih.gov/books/NBK8191/

[3] Postigo I, Guisantes JA, Martínez J. Is there a link between environmental allergens and parasitism? In: Kon K, Rai M, editors. The Microbiology of Respiratory System Infections. London, UK: Academic Press; 2016. pp. 113-124

[4] Husain MA, Scheibel LW. Anthelmintic drugs. In: Craig CR, Stitzel RE, editors. Modern Pharmacology with Clinical Applications. 5th ed. Philadelphia, PA: Lippincott Williams & Wilkins; 2004. pp. 348-354

[5] World Health Organization. Guideline: Preventive Chemotherapy to Control Soil-Transmitted Helminth Infections in At-Risk Population Groups. Geneva, Swizerland: World Health Organization; 2017

[6] Khan PR, Karthikeyan M, Kannan M, Rajasekar S. Anthelmintic activity of *Nerium olender* flower extract in Indian adult earthworm. Journal of Natural Product and Plant Resources. 2011;**1**(4):40-46

[7] Adate PS, Parmesawaran S, Chauhan Y. In vitro anthelmintic activity of stem extracts of *Piper betle* Linn against *Pheretima posthuman*. Pharmacognosy Journal. 2012;**4**(29):61-65

[8] Boddupally SR, Edula V, Nagulu M. Evaluation of antibacterial and antihelminthic activity of polyherbal gel. World Journal of Pharmaceutical Research. 2018;**7**(05):1346-1354

[9] Debebe Y, Tefera M, Mekonnen W, Abebe D, Woldekidan S, Abebe A, et al. Evaluation of anthelmintic potential of the Ethiopian medicinal plant *Embelia schimperi* Vatke *in vivo* and *in vitro* against some intestinal parasites. Complementary and Alternative Medicine. 2015;**15**(1):1-6

[10] Tagboto S, Townson S. Antiparasitic properties of medicinal plants and other naturally occurring products. Advances in Parasitology. 2001;**50**:199-295

[11] Kumar PS. *In-Vitro* antihelminthic activity, photo chemical screening and TLC studies of methanol extraction on *Celosia Cristata* flower using in – State festival of Telangana (Bathukamma). World Journal of Pharmaceutical Research. 2018;**7**(7):1073-1086

[12] World Health Organization. Ending the Neglect to Attain the Sustainable Development Goals: A Road Map for Neglected Tropical Diseases 2021-2030. Geneva, Swizerland: World Health Organization; 2020

[13] Awasthi S, Bundy DA, Savioli L. Helminthic infections. British Media Journal. 2003;**327**(7412):431-433

[14] King CH. Health metrics for helminthic infections. Advances in Parasitology. 2010;**1**(73):51-69

[15] Loukas A, Maizels RM, Hotez PJ. The Yin and Yang of human soil-transmitted helminth infections.

International Journal for Parasitology. 2022;**51**(13-14):1243-1253

[16] Kumarasingha R, Preston S, Yeo TC, Lim DSL, Tu CL, Palombo EA, et al. Anthelmintic activity of selected ethno-medicinal plant extracts on parasitic stages of *Haemonchus contortus*. Parasites & Vectors. 2016;**9**(1):1-7

[17] Sori T, Bekana M, Adunga G, Kelbesa E. Medicinal plants in ethnoveterinary practices of Borana pastoralists, Southern Ethiopia. International Journal of Applied Research in Veterinary Medicine. 2004;**2**(3):220-225

[18] Getachew S, Ibrahim N, Abebe B, Eguale T. *In vitro* evaluation of anthelmintic activities of crude extracts of selected medicinal plants against *Haemonchus contortus* in Alemgena Wereda, Ethiopia. Acta Parasitologica Globalis. 2012;**3**(2):20-27

[19] Lambert SM, Nishi SM, Mendonça LR, da Silva Souza BMP, da Silva JF, da Silva GP, et al. Genotypic profile of benzimidazole resistance associated with SNP F167Y and F200Y Beta-Tubulin Gene in Brazilian populations of *Haemonchus contortus* of goats. Veterinary Parasitology: Regional Studies and Reports. 2017;**8**:28-34

[20] Waller PJ. Sustainable helminth control of ruminants in developing countries. Veterinary Parasitology. 1997;**71**(2-3):195-207

[21] Ogbaje CI, Agbo EO, Ajanusi OJ. Prevalence of *Ascaridia galli*, *Heterakis gallinarum* and tapeworm infections in birds slaughtered in Makurdi Township. International Journal of Poultry Science. 2012;**11**(2):103-107

[22] Matthews JB. Facing the threat of equine parasitic disease. Equine Veterinary Journal. 2011;**43**(2):126-132

[23] Scantlebury CE, Peachey L, Hodgkinson Jmatthews JB, Trawford A, Mulugeta G, Tefera G, et al. Participatory study of medicinal plants used in the control of gastrointestinal parasites in donkeys in eastern Shewa and Arsi Zones of Oromia Region, Ethiopia. Veterinary Research. 2013;**9**(1):179

[24] Jia-Chi C, Abdullah NA, Shukor N, Jaturas N, Richard RL, Abd Majid MA, et al. Soil transmitted helminths in animals–How is it possible for human transmission? Asian Pacific Journal of Tropical Disease. 2016;**6**(11):859-863

[25] Al Amin ASM, Wadhwa R. Helminthiasis. Treasure Island, FL: StatPearls Publishing; 2020

[26] Albonico M, Crompton DWT, Savioli L. Control strategies for human intestinal nematode infections. Advances in Parasitology. 1999;**42**:277-341

[27] Jourdan PM, Lamberton PH, Fenwick A, Addiss DG. Soil-transmitted helminth infections. The Lancet. 2018;**391**(10117):252-265

[28] Bethony J, Brooker S, Albonico M, Geiger SM, Loukas A, Diemert D, et al. (2006). Soil-transmitted helminth infections: *Ascariasis, Trichuriasis, and Hookworm*. The Lancet. 2006;**367**(9521):1521-1532

[29] Bansal Y, Silakari O. The therapeutic journey of Benzimidazoles: A review. Bioorganic & Medicinal Chemistry. 2012;**20**(21):6208-6236

[30] Keri RS, Hiremathad A, Budagumpi S, Nagaraja BM. Comprehensive review in current developments of benzimidazole-based medicinal chemistry. Chemical Biology & Drug Design. 2014, 2014;**86**(1):19-65

[31] Yadav G, Ganguly S. Structure activity relationship (SAR) study of

benzimidazole scaffold for different biological activities: A mini-review. European Journal of Medicinal Chemistry. 2015;**2015**(97):419-443

[32] Shaharyar M, Mazumder A. Benzimidazoles: A biologically active compounds. Arabian Journal of Chemistry. 2017;**10**:S157-S173

[33] Brown HD, Matzuk AR, Ilves I, Peterson LH, Harris SA, Sarett LH, et al. 2-(4′-thiazolyl)-benzimidazole, a new anthelmintic. Journal of the American Chemical Society. 1961;**83**(7):1764-1765

[34] Townsend LB, Wise DS. The synthesis and chemistry of certain anthelmintic benzimidazoles. Parasitology Today. 1990;**6**(4):107-112

[35] Sharma S, Abuzar S. The benzimidazole anthelmintics—chemistry and biological activity. In: Progress in Drug Research/Fortschritte der Arzneimittelforschung/Progrès des recherches pharmaceutiques. 1983. pp. 85-161

[36] Lacey E. The role of the cytoskeletal protein, tubulin, in the mode of action and mechanism of drug resistance to benzimidazoles. International Journal for Parasitology. 1988;**18**(7):885-936

[37] Lacey E. Mode of action of benzimidazoles. Parasitology Today. 1990;**6**(4):112-115

[38] Amery WK, Bruynseels JP. Levamisole, the story and the lessons. International Journal of Immunopharmacology. 1992;**14**(3):481-486

[39] Köhler P. The biochemical basis of anthelmintic action and resistance. International Journal for Parasitology. 2001;**31**(4):336-345

[40] Yadav P, Singh R. A review on anthelmintic drugs and their future scope. International Journal of Pharmacy and Pharmaceutical Sciences. 2011;**3**(3):17-21

[41] Holden-Dye L, Walker R. Anthelmintic drugs and nematocides: Studies in *Caenorhabditis elegans*. WormBook: The Online Review of C. elegans Biology. 2014:1-29

[42] Sheehan DJ, Sheehan SM, Marchiondo AA. Discovery and chemistry of Pyrantel, Morantel and Oxantel. In: Pyrantel Parasiticide Therapy in Humans and Domestic Animals. Academic Press; 2016. pp. 1-19

[43] Aubry ML, Cowell P, Davey MJ, Shevde S. Aspects of the pharmacology of a new anthelmintic: Pyrantel. British Journal of Pharmacology. 1970;**38**(2):332-344

[44] Martin RJ, Robertson AP, Choudhary S. Ivermectin: An anthelmintic, an insecticide, and much more. Trends in Parasitology. 2021;**37**(1):48-64

[45] Enejoh OS, Suleiman MM. Anthelmintics and their application in veterinary medicine. Research in Medical and Engineering Sciences. 2017;**2**(3)

[46] Geary TG, Moreno Y. Macrocyclic lactone anthelmintics: Spectrum of activity and mechanism of action. Current Pharmaceutical Biotechnology. 2012;**13**(6):866-872

[47] Austin WC, Courtney W, Danilewicz JC, Morgan DH, Conover LH, Howes HJ, et al. Pyrantel tartrate, a new anthelmintic effective against infections of domestic animals. Nature. 1966;**212**(5067):1273-1274

[48] Magiliny S, Murugananthan A, Kannathasan S, and Silva NRD. First

report on the *in vitro* anthelmintic activity of *Centella Asiatica* ("Gotu Kola"/"Vallarai"). In: Proceedings of 8th International Research Conference, KDU. 2015. pp. 57-59

[49] Naidu KN, Ramu DV, Kumar NSS. Anti-inflammatory and anti-helminthic activity of ethanolic extract of *Azadirachta indica* leaves. International Journal of Green Pharmacy. 2016;**10**(4):200-203

[50] Sepúlveda-Crespo D, Reguera RM, Rojo-Vázquez F, Balaña-Fouce R, Martínez-Valladares M. Drug discovery technologies: *Caenorhabditis elegans* as a model for anthelmintic therapeutics. Medicinal Research Reviews. 2020;**40**(5):1715-1753

[51] Wolstenholme AJ, Martin RJ. Anthelmintics–from discovery to resistance. International Journal for Parasitology: Drugs and Drug Resistance. 2014;**4**(3):218-219

[52] World Health Organization. Preventive Chemotherapy in Human Helminthiasis. World Health Organization; 2006

[53] Zajíčková M, Nguyen LT, Skálová L, Stuchlíková LR, Matoušková P. Anthelmintics in the future: Current trends in the discovery and development of new drugs against gastrointestinal nematodes. Drug Discovery Today. 2020;**25**(2):430-437

[54] Nixon SA, Welz C, Woods DJ, Costa-Junior L, Zamanian M, Martin RJ. Where are all the anthelmintics? Challenges and opportunities on the path to new anthelmintics. International Journal for Parasitology: Drugs and Drug Resistance. 2020;**14**:8-16

[55] Jayawardene KLT, Palombo EA, Boag PR. Natural products are a promising source for anthelmintic drug discovery. Biomolecules. 2021, 2021;**11**(10):1457

[56] Atanasov AG, Waltenberger B, Pferschy-WenzigEM,LinderT,WawroschC, Uhrin P, et al. Discovery and resupply of pharmacologically active plant-derived natural products: A review. Biotechnology Advances. 2015;**33**(8):1582-1614

[57] Herath HD, Taki AC, Sleebs BE, Hofmann A, Nguyen N, Preston S, et al. Advances in the discovery and development of anthelmintics by harnessing natural product scaffolds. Advances in Parasitology. 2021;**111**:203-251

[58] Herath HD, Preston S, Jabbar A, Garcia-Bustos J, Addison RS, Hayes S, et al. Selected α-pyrones from the Plants *Cryptocarya novoguineensis* (Lauraceae) and *Piper methysticum* (Piperaceae) with Activity Against *Haemonchus contortus in vitro*. International Journal for Parasitology: Drugs and Drug Resistance. 2019;**9**:72-79

[59] Herath HD, Taki AC, Nguyen N, Garcia-Bustos J, Hofmann A, Wang T, et al. Synthetic kavalactone analogues with increased potency and selective anthelmintic activity against larvae of *Haemonchus contortus in vitro*. Molecules. 2020;**25**(8):2004

[60] Herath HD, Preston S, Jabbar A, Garcia-Bustos J, Taki AC, Addison RS, et al. Identification of Fromiamycalin and Halaminol a from Australian marine sponge extracts with anthelmintic activity against *Haemonchus Contortus*. Marine Drugs. 2019;**17**(11):598

[61] Farrugia M, Trotter N, Vijayasarathy S, Salim AA, Khalil ZG, Lacey E, et al. Isolation and synthesis of N-Acyladenine and adenosine alkaloids from a Southern Australian marine

sponge, *Phoriospongia* sp. Tetrahedron Letters. 2014;**55**(43):5902-5904

[62] Capon RJ, Vuong D, McNally M, Peterle T, Trotter N, Lacey E, et al. (+)-Echinobetaine B: Isolation, structure elucidation, synthesis and preliminary SAR studies on a new nematocidal betaine from a Southern Australian Marine Sponge, *Echinodictyum* sp. Organic & Biomolecular Chemistry. 2005;**3**(1):118-122

[63] Zajíčková M, Prchal L, Vokřál I, Nguyen LT, Kurz T, Gasser R, et al. Assessing the anthelmintic candidates BLK127 and HBK4 for their efficacy on *Haemonchus contortus* adults and eggs, and their hepatotoxicity and biotransformation. Pharmaceutics. 2022;**14**(4):754

[64] Burns AR, Luciani GM, Musso G, Bagg R, Yeo M, Zhang Y, et al. Caenorhabditis elegans is a useful model for anthelmintic discovery. Nature Communications. 2015;**6**(1):1-11

[65] Mathew MD, Mathew ND, Miller A, Simpson M, Au V, Garland S, et al. Using *C. elegans* forward and reverse genetics to identify new compounds with anthelmintic activity. PLoS Neglected Tropical Diseases. 2016;**10**(10):e0005058

[66] Vairoletti F, Paulino M, Mahler G, Salinas G, Saiz C. Structure-based bioisosterism design, synthesis, biological evaluation and in silico studies of benzamide analogs as potential anthelmintics. Molecules. 2022;**27**(9):2659

[67] Preston S, Jiao Y, Baell JB, Keiser J, Crawford S, Koehler AV, et al. Screening of the "open scaffolds" collection from compounds Australia identifies a new chemical entity with anthelmintic activities against different developmental stages of the barber's pole worm and other parasitic nematodes. International Journal for Parasitology: Drugs and Drug Resistance. 2017;**7**(3):286-294

[68] Le TG, Kundu A, Ghoshal A, Nguyen NH, Preston S, Jiao Y, et al. Optimization Of Novel 1-Methyl-1 H-Pyrazole-5-carboxamides leads to high potency larval development inhibitors of the barber's pole worm. Journal of Medicinal Chemistry. 2018;**61**(23):10875-10894

[69] Le TG, Kundu A, Ghoshal A, Nguyen NH, Preston S, Jiao Y, et al. Novel 1-Methyl-1 H-Pyrazole-5-carboxamide derivatives with potent anthelmintic activity. Journal of Medicinal Chemistry. 2019;**62**(7):3367-3380

[70] Ruan B, Zhang Y, Tadesse S, Preston S, Taki AC, Jabbar A, et al. Synthesis and structure-activity relationship study of pyrrolidine-oxadiazoles as anthelmintics against *Haemonchus Contortus*. European Journal of Medicinal Chemistry. 2020;**190**:112100

[71] Nguyen LT, Kurz T, Preston S, Brueckmann H, Lungerich B, Herath HM, et al. Phenotypic screening of the "Kurz-Box" of chemicals identifies two compounds (BLK127 and HBK4) with anthelmintic activity *in vitro* against parasitic larval stages of *Haemonchus contortus*. Parasites & Vectors. 2019;**12**(1):1-9

[72] Risi G, Aguilera E, Ladós E, Suárez G, Carrera I, Álvarez G, et al. *Caenorhabditis elegans* infrared-based motility assay identified new hits for nematicide drug development. Veterinary Sciences. 2019;**6**(1):29

[73] Partridge FA, Forman R, Willis NJ, Bataille CJ, Murphy EA, Brown AE, et al. 2, 4-Diaminothieno [3, 2-d] pyrimidines, a new class of anthelmintic with activity against adult and egg stages

of whipworm. PLoS Neglected Tropical Diseases. 2018;**12**(7):e0006487

[74] Partridge FA, Murphy EA, Willis NJ, Bataille CJ, Forman R, Heyer-Chauhan N, et al. Dihydrobenz [e][1, 4] oxazepin-2 (3 H)-ones, a new anthelmintic chemotype immobilising whipworm and reducing infectivity *in vivo*. PLoS Neglected Tropical Diseases. 2017;**11**(2):e0005359

[75] Partridge FA, Bataille CJ, Forman R, Marriott AE, Forde-Thomas J, Häberli C, et al. Structural requirements for dihydrobenzoxazepinone anthelmintics: Actions against medically important and model parasites: *Trichuris muris, Brugia malayi, Heligmosomoides polygyrus*, and *Schistosoma mansoni*. ACS Infectious Diseases. 2021;**7**(5):1260-1274

[76] Rossiter S, Peron JM, Whitfield PJ, Jones K. Synthesis and anthelmintic properties of arylquinolines with activity against drug-resistant nematodes. Bioorganic & Medicinal Chemistry Letters. 2005;**15**(21):4806-4808

[77] Milišiūnaitė V, Kadlecová A, Žukauskaitė A, Doležal K, Strnad M, Voller J, et al. Synthesis and anthelmintic activity of benzopyrano [2, 3-c] pyrazol-4 (2H)-one derivatives. Molecular Diversity. 2020;**24**(4):1025-1042

[78] Pushpakom S, Iorio F, Eyers PA, Escott KJ, Hopper S, Wells A, et al. Drug repurposing: Progress, challenges and recommendations. Nature Reviews. Drug Discovery. 2019;**18**(1):41-58

[79] Sekhon BS. Repositioning drugs and biologics: Retargeting old/existing drugs for potential new therapeutic applications. Journal of Pharmaceutical Education & Research. 2013 Jun;**4**(1)

[80] Panic G, Duthaler U, Speich B, Keiser J. Repurposing drugs for the treatment and control of helminth infections. International Journal for Parasitology: Drugs and Drug Resistance. 2014;**4**(3):185-200

[81] Krücken J, Harder A, Jeschke P, Holden-Dye L, O'Connor V, Welz C, et al. Anthelmintic cyclooctadepsipeptides: Complex in structure and mode of action. Trends in Parasitology. 2012;**28**(9):385-394

[82] von Samson-Himmelstjerna G, Harder A, Sangster NC, Coles GC. Efficacy of two cyclooctadepsipeptides, PF1022A and emodepside, against anthelmintic-resistant nematodes in sheep and cattle. Parasitology. 2005;**130**(3):343-347

[83] Sasaki T, Takagi M, Yaguchi T, Miyadoh S, Okada T, Koyama M. A new anthelminticcyclodepsipeptide,PF1022A. The Journal of Antibiotics. 1992;**45**(5):692-697

[84] Scherkenbeck J, Jeschke P, Harder A. PF1022A and related cyclodepsipeptides - A novel class of anthelmintics. Current Topics in Medicinal Chemistry. 2002;**2**(7):759-777

[85] Karpstein T, Pasche V, Häberli C, Scandale I, Neodo A, Keiser J. Evaluation of emodepside in laboratory models of human intestinal nematode and schistosome infections. Parasites & Vectors. 2019;**12**(1):1

[86] Sivanathan S, Körber F, Scherkenbeck J. Semisynthetic routes to PF1022H—A precursor for new derivatives of the anthelmintic cyclooctadepsipeptide PF1022A. Bioorganic & Medicinal Chemistry. 2016;**24**(4):873-876

[87] Weeks JC, Roberts WM, Leasure C, Suzuki BM, Robinson KJ, Currey H, et al. Sertraline, paroxetine,

and chlorpromazine are rapidly acting anthelmintic drugs capable of clinical repurposing. Scientific Reports. 2018;**8**(1):1-7

[88] Jiao Y, Preston S, Koehler AV, Stroehlein AJ, Chang BC, Simpson KJ, et al. Screening of the "Stasis Box" identifies two kinase inhibitors under pharmaceutical development with activity against *Haemonchus contortus*. Parasites & Vectors. 2017;**10**(1):1-7

[89] Jiao Y, Preston S, Garcia-Bustos JF, Baell JB, Ventura S, Le T, et al. Tetrahydroquinoxalines induce a lethal evisceration phenotype in *Haemonchus contortus in vitro*. International Journal for Parasitology: Drugs and Drug Resistance. 2019;**9**:59-71

[90] Campos N, Myburgh R, Garcel A, Vautrin A, Lapasset L, Nadal ES, et al. Long lasting control of viral rebound with a new drug ABX464 targeting rev–mediated viral RNA biogenesis. Retrovirology. 2015;**12**(1):1-5

[91] Shanley HT, Taki AC, Byrne JJ, Jabbar A, Wells TN, Samby K, et al. A high-throughput phenotypic screen of the "pandemic response box" identifies a quinoline derivative with significant anthelmintic activity. Pharmaceuticals. 2022;**15**(2):257

[92] Liu M, Landuyt B, Klaassen H, Geldhof P, Luyten W. Screening of a drug repurposing library with a nematode motility assay identifies promising anthelmintic hits against *Cooperia oncophora* and other ruminant parasites. Veterinary Parasitology. 2019;**265**:15-18

[93] Keiser J, Panic G, Adelfio R, Cowan N, Vargas M, Scandale I. Evaluation of an FDA approved library against laboratory models of human intestinal nematode infections. Parasites & Vectors. 2016;**9**(1):1

[94] Herath HD, Song H, Preston S, Jabbar A, Wang T, McGee SL, et al. Arylpyrrole and fipronil analogues that inhibit the motility and/or development of *Haemonchus contortus in vitro*. International Journal for Parasitology: Drugs and Drug Resistance. 2018;**8**(3):379-385

[95] Pattanayak P, Kaliyaperumal S. Design, synthesis, characterization and *in vitro* antimicrobial and anthelmintic evaluation of metronidazole derivatives modified at position 1. Pharmaceutical Chemistry Journal. 2022;**56**(2):191-196

[96] Munguía B, Saldaña J, Nieves M, Melian ME, Ferrer M, Teixeira R, et al. Sensitivity of *Haemonchus contortus* to anthelmintics using different *in vitro* screening assays: A comparative study. Parasites & Vectors. 2022;**15**(1):1

[97] Sethi P, Bansal Y, Bansal G. Synthesis and PASS-assisted evaluation of coumarin–benzimidazole derivatives as potential anti-inflammatory and anthelmintic agents. Medicinal Chemistry Research. 2018;**27**(1):61-71

[98] Lin Y, Ong YC, Keller S, Karges J, Bouchene R, Manoury E, et al. Synthesis, characterization and antiparasitic activity of organometallic derivatives of the anthelmintic drug albendazole. Dalton Transactions. 2020;**49**(20):6616-6626

[99] Huang J, Chen AL, Zhang H, Yu Z, Li MH, Li N, et al. Gene replacement for the generation of designed novel avermectin derivatives with enhanced acaricidal and nematicidal activities. Applied and Environmental Microbiology. 2015;**81**(16):5326-5334

[100] Fei C, She R, Li G, Zhang L, Fan W, Xue F. Safety and clinical efficacy of tenvermectin, a novel antiparasitic 16-membered macrocyclic lactone

antibiotics. European Journal of Pharmaceutical Sciences. 2018;**117**:154-160

[101] Keiser J, Tritten L, Silberesien A, Speich B, Adelfio R, Vargas M. Activity of oxantel pamoate monotherapy and combination chemotherapy against *Trichuris muris* and hookworms: revival of an old drug. PLoS Neglected Tropical Diseases. 2013;**7**(3):e2119

[102] Moser W, Sayasone S, Xayavong S, Bounheuang B, Puchkov M, Huwyler J, et al. Efficacy and tolerability of triple drug therapy with albendazole, pyrantel pamoate, and oxantel pamoate compared with albendazole plus oxantel pamoate, pyrantel pamoate plus oxantel pamoate, and mebendazole plus pyrantel pamoate and oxantel pamoate against hookworm infections in school-aged children in Laos: a randomised, single-blind trial. The Lancet. 2018;**18**(7):729-737

[103] Zawawi A, Forman R, Smith H, Mair I, Jibril M, Albaqshi MH, et al. *In Silico* Design of a T-Cell Epitope Vaccine Candidate for Parasitic Helminth Infection. PLoS Pathogens. 2020;**16**(3):e1008243

[104] Diemert DJ, Bottazzi ME, Plieskatt J, Hotez PJ, Bethony JM. Lessons Along The Critical Path: Developing Vaccines Against Human Helminths. Trends in Parasitology. 2018;**34**(9): 747-758

[105] Zawawi A, Else KJ. Soil-transmitted helminth vaccines: are we getting closer? Frontiers in Immunology. 2020;**11**:576748

[106] Zhan B, Beaumier CM, Briggs N, Jones KM, Keegan BP, Bottazzi ME, et al. Advancing a Multivalent "Pan-Anthelmintic" Vaccine Against Soil-Transmitted Nematode Infections. Expert Review of Vaccines. 2014;**13**(3):321-331

Chapter 4

Evaluation, Diagnosis and Treatment of *Ascariasis*: An Updated Review

Narendra Nath Mukhopadhyay

Abstract

Ascaris lumbricoides (Round Worm) is the most common human helminth with a world wide distribution. Incidence of ascariasis remain very high in the tropical and sub tropical countries with poor sanitation, personal hygiene, and rural areas where defaecation in open place is still a common practice. Ascariasis is classified as a neglected tropical disease. Infections have no symptoms in more than 85 percent of cases specially if the number of cases are small. Pathogenecity and clinical features are either due to migrating larvae or due to adult worms. Larval migration may lead to allergic reactions, ascaris pneumonia. Adult worms are often responsible for nutritional deficiencies, toxic effects due to hypersensitivity &mechanical effects leading to intestinal obstruction. Ectopic ascariasis can lead to acute biliary obstruction, cholangitis, acute pancreatitis, acute obstructive appendicitis and peritonitis due to perforation of an intestinal ulcer or break down of a post operative suture line. Medical therapy with Albendazole is the first line drug ascariasis can be eliminated by preventing faecal contamination of soil. Advancement in recombinant protein technology may provide first step in discovery of Ascaris vaccine as well as pan helminthic Vaccine. This chapter is a updated review of ascariasis.

Keywords: *ascariasis*, round worm, human helminth

1. Introduction

GENUS: *Ascaris lumbricoides Linnaeus 1758*

Species: *A. lumbricoides*

The common roundworm

The study was conducted analysing the inputs from various articles presented with general description of *Ascaris lumbricoides* and study results were analysed.

Cram in 1926 mentioned the hookworm and the malarial parasite have been the objects of international campaign of far reaching scope while the ascarid has received only causal attention. And yet this parasite is of very great importance because it is so wide spread and the pathological effect on the individual may be so very serious.

Ascaris lumbricoides, a soil transmitted helminth is the largest nematode infecting human with a worldwide distribution. The nematodes are unsegmented ones. They are elongated and cylindrical with tapering ends.

The specific name lumbricoides is derived from its resemblance to earthworm (in Latin lumbricoides meaning earthworm).

Ascaris has been described from very ancient times. It was described in Egyptian papyrus and found in Egyptian mummies. This helminth has been described by Hippocrates and Aristotle. About 0.8 to 1.2 billion people around the world are infected with ascaris. It is more common in tropical and sub tropical countries around the world and most heavily affected population being in the sub Saharan Africa [1–3], Latin America, China and East Asia with poor sanitation, poor personal hygiene and places where defecation in open place is common practice.

Ascaris is classified as a neglected tropical disease [4–6].

Infections have no symptoms in more than 85% of the cases specially if the numbers of worms are small.

Children are most commonly affected [7]. Because of its global presence and potential to cause severe morbidity and mortality ascaris must be considered as a major health hazard.

Its global distribution is so high an editorial in Lancet in 1989 observed that if all the roundworms in the entire affected individual worldwide were placed end to end then they can encircle the world 50 times.

A species- Ascaris sum morphologically identical but biologically separate which is a pig roundworm rarely infect human being. It is unknown how many people are infected with ascaris sum worldwide.

2. Habitat

The adult worm lives in the lumen of small intestine (85% in jejunum [1, 8], and 15% in ileum) and maintain its position by muscle tone. Ascaris takes most of its nutrients from the partially digested food in the intestine. They can secrete inhibitory enzymes to protect itself from digestion by host's enzymes. Adult worm survive for 1 to 2 years in human host after which it dies and spontaneously evacuated from the digestive tract.

3. Morphology

Adult worm– Largest intestinal nematode resembles an ordinary earthworm. When fresh from the intestine it is pale pink or light brown in colour but become white outside the body. The mouth opens at the anterior end and possesses three finely toothed lips- one dorsal and two ventral.

Male worm – It is 15 to 25 cm in length with a diameter of 3 to 4 mm. The tail end is curved ventrally to form a hook. The genital pore opens into the cloacae and carries two copulatory spicules.

Female worm- It is longer than male and measures 25 to 40 cm with a diameter of 3 to 6 mm. posterior end is straight and conical. The vulva opens at the junction of anterior and middle third of the body and this section is narrower and is called the vulval waist. A mature female worm lays up to 2,00,000 eggs per day. The eggs are passed in the faeces.

Eggs- Eggs can be fertilised or unfertilized.

a. Fertilised egg- Round or oval in shape, always bile stained. Fertilised eggs are embryonated and develop into infective eggs.

b. Unfertilized eggs- Narrower, longer, brownish in colour. They are non embyonated and non infective.

Both fertilised and unfertilized eggs may be found in a sample of stool or either type alone. Specimens showing only the unfertilized eggs signify that the host is harbouring only female worm.

4. Lifecycle

Man is the only natural host and there is no intermediate host. Lifecycle of the parasite were not known before 1916.

INFECTIVE AGENT – Embryonated eggs.

Mode of transmission – Infection occurs when embryonated eggs are swallowed with contaminated food and water.

Stage 1- Fertilised eggs containing the unsegmented ovum are passed with the feceas. They are not immediately infective.

Stage 2- Development in soil- under suitable climatic condition of temperature 25 to 30 degree centigrade, high humidity, and adequate oxygen supply fertilised eggs mault once and rhabtidiform larvae developed from the unsegmented worm within the egg cell in 10 to 40 days time. The fertilised egg of Ascaris is the most resistant and can remain viable in the hostile environment for many years.

Stage 3- Swallowing of infective eggs and liberation of larvae.

The swallowed eggs passed down to duodenum where egg shell weakened by the digestive juice and rhabtidiform larva about 250 microns in length and 14 micron in diameter liberated in upper part of small intestine.

Stage 4- Migration through the lungs.

The larvae penetrate the intestinal mucosa and enter the portal circulation and carried to liver. From liver it passes via the hepatic veins, Inferior vena cava and right side of the heart to the lungs in about 4 days. In the lungs they grow much bigger and moult twice. Subsequently they penetrate the capillary wall and enter the lung alveoli in about 10 to 15 days.

Stage 5- Re-entry into the small intestine.

From the lung alveoli the larvae pass up the bronchi and trachea, where they are coughed up and may be swallowed. The larvae pass down the oesophagus to the stomach and reach the upper part of small intestine- their normal habitat.

Stage 6- Maturity.

The larvae on reaching their habitat grow into adult worm. They become sexually mature in about 6 to 12 weeks time. The gravid female start laying eggs which is passed in the stool and the cycle is repeated [9, 10].

5. Clinical manifestations

5.1 Symptoms due to migrating larvae

Ascaris pneumonia (Loeffler's syndrome) – Pulmonary manifestations take place during larval migration and characterised by low grade fever, cough, dyspnoea, urticaria and eosinophilia.

The sputum is often blood stained and may contain Charcot- layden crystals.

Chest x-ray may show pulmonary infiltrate with radiographic shadowing.

The larvae may be found in sputum and more often in gastric washing. This pneumonia usually clears up in 1 to2 weeks but sometimes may be severe [8, 11]. Ascaris induced eosinophilic myocarditis have been reported in literature [12].

5.2 Symptoms due to adult worm

1. *Nutritional deficiency*: *Ascaris lumbricoides* induces changes in the jejunal mucosal and intestinal muscle layers. There is coarsening of mucosa folds, crypt depth shortening, reduced mucus production and hypertrophy of muscle layers [13, 14].

   Where large numbers of worms are present specially in children interfere with proper digestion and absorption of food and can lead to protein energy malnutrition, vitamin A deficiency and impaired cognitive function in children [15].

2. *Toxic effects:* Hypersensitivity to Ascaris antigen can lead to fever, urticaria, Angioneurotic oedema, conjunctivitis.

3. *Mechanical effects:* This is the most important manifestation of Ascariasis. Bowel obstruction may occur in upto 0.2 per 1000 per year [7]. When large numbers of worms get strangled into a bolus may lead to luminal occlusion and acute intestinal obstruction [16–18]. Perforation may occur due to ischemic pressure necrosis by roundworm ball. It can precipitate intussusceptions, volvulus and closed loop obstruction. It may perforate through any ulcer of the alimentary tract and can lead to peritonitis. Free lying ascaris can be seen floating in the peritoneal cavity. We have reported a case of duodeno ureteric fistula caused by ascaris [19].

4. *Ectopic Ascariasis:* Migration is a common habit of ascaris. Fever, ingestion of some drugs and foods by the host and surgical anaesthesia is a predisposing factor for worm migration from its natural location. Going up it may pass through the oesophagus and coming out through mouth or nose. It may enter the trachea causing respiratory obstruction. Rarely it may enter the biliary or pancreatic duct causing obstructive jaundice, cholangitis, acute pancreatitis and liver abscess. Going down worm may enter the appendix giving rise to acute obstructive appendicitis [9, 10, 20–22]. In gastrointestinal surgery requiring resection and anastomosis it may perforate through the suture line. So in endemic areas it is recommended pre-operative deworming before gastrointestinal surgery.

DOI: http://dx.doi.org/10.5772/intechopen.109147

6. Diagnosis

a. *Direct evidence:*

Larvae: During the pulmonary disease larvae may be found in sputum or more often in gastric juice. Findings of Charcot – layden crystal in sputum and eosinophilia may further help in the diagnosis.

Eggs: The best diagnostic test is still the stool examination demonstrating eggs as the Ascaris eggs are passed in stool in enormous numbers. It is easy to detect the affected person by direct microscopical examination of a saline emulsion of the stool.

It is important to note that stool can be negative while the worm migrates and matures. Both fertilised and unfertilized eggs may be present, occasionally only one type is seen. If the patient harbours male ascaris only, eggs are not found in the stool.

Microscopical examination of bile obtained by duodenal aspirate may reveal ascaris eggs. Eggs in the biliary tree can act as a nidus for stone formation.

Adult worms: Occasional findings of adult worm in stool and vomit.

b. *Serological tests:* Detection of Ascaris antibody by indirect hemagglutination and ELISA test.

c. *Blood examination:* Eosinophilia in early stage of infection.

d. *Imaging:*

X-ray Abdomen: Bolus of worms may be found with whirled appearance (whirlpool sign) in intestinal obstruction.

Barium Meal Follow through: Round worm may be identified with barium within.

CECT Abdomen: may show curvilinear structure within the lumen of intestine.

USG and MRCP: may demonstrate worm in CBD and pancreatic duct in the setting of obstructive jaundice, acute cholangitis, and acute pancreatitis.

7. Treatment/management:

a. *PREVENTION* – Ascaris can be eliminated by preventing faecal contamination of soil. Improved access to sanitation, prohibition of open defecation, use of clean toilet by all community members, provision of clean drinking water, maintenance of general hygiene and health education, avoiding of untreated human fecaes as fertiliser will help in reducing ascsaris egg contamination.

Washing of vegetables with water containing iodine 200 PPM for 15 minutes kills the eggs of Ascaris and other helminth.
In areas where more than 20% of population is affected treating the whole community with deworming agent is recommended as prophylaxis [7]. This is known as Mass drug administration and targeted population specially at the school age children [23]. As recommended by WHO, drug of choice is Albendazole or Mebendazole.

b. *Medications* – To prevent serious complications even mild cases of ascariasis should be treated with proper medications. Those recommended by WHO for ascariasis are Albendazole, Mebendazole, Levamisole and Pyrantal pamoate [24].

Medical therapy with albendazole 400 mg as a single dose is the first line of drug. Second choice is mebendazole 100 mg twice a day for 3 days or 500 mg as a single dose or Ivermectin 100 microgram per kg to 200 microgram per kg once [25].
The major site of action of albendazole and mebendazole is the microtubular protein *"Beta Tubulin"* of the worm. It binds to the *beta tubulin* of the worm with high affinity and inhibits its polymerisation. Intracellular microtubules in the cells of the parasite lost. It blocks glucose uptake by the parasite. Hatching of nematode eggs and their larvae are also inhibited. Ascaris ova are also killed. Albendazole is contraindicated during pregnancy and children less than 2 years of age.
Pyrantal pamoate: Pyrantal activates nicotinic cholinergic receptors in the worm causing spastic paralysis. Worms are then expelled. For Ascaris single dose of 11 mg/kg is recommended. Pyrantal may induce intestinal obstruction in the presence of heavy worm load. It can be used in pregnancy.
Piparazine: It causes flaccid paralysis of the worm and worms are expelled alive by peristalsis. Often a purgative is given with it. Because of its ability to relax ascaris it is of particular value in intestinal obstruction due to roundworm. It can be used during pregnancy.
Other medications:
Nitazoxanide
Hexylresorcinol
Ivermectin
Levamisole
Tetramisole
Children should receive Vitamin A supplementation because of vitamin A deficiency in ascasriasis. Retreatment in 3 to 6 months is recommended in endemic areas.

c. *Vaccine*: There is a significant challenge to control and eradicate ascariasis especially in endemic areas. Mass drug administration programme with benzimidazole anti-helminthics are the only methods available to control infection. Ascaris eggs are highly resistant in adverse environment which limit the ability of mass drug administration to break the transmission cycle in the community. So post treatment reinfection is common. Besides frequent anti-helminthic administration may result in complications including development of drug resistance. So only solution to eradicate the disease globally is vaccination against ascariasis. However till date no effective vaccine available for human clinical trial. Advancement in recombinant protein technology may provide the first step in generating an ascaris vaccine as well as pan-helminthic vaccine [26].

d. Surgery: In sub acute intestinal obstruction, conservative treatment in the form of IV fluid, NG suction and hypertonic saline enema is recommended.

Hypertonic saline enema disimpact the roundworm bolus and stimulates intestinal peristalsis. Operation is required for acute intestinal obstruction and perforation.
During laparotomy, attempt should be made to milk the ascaris mass to the colon through ileo-caecal valve for natural evacuation.
In healthy bowel, enterotomy and removal of round worm bolus may be required.
Perforation, gangrene require resection and anstomosis.
In perforation it is safe to exteriorize the perforation site as ileostomy because chances of suture line breakdown due to roundworm activity are increased.
Sometimes roundworms may be an incidental finding in typhoid perforation, tuberculosis, and other causes of intestinal obstruction.
Post operative deworming is always necessary to kill the residual egg.
ERCP – In Pancreaticobiliary ascariasis ERCP may be both diagnostic and therapeutic [27].

8. Present review result shows

1. Ascaris is the commonest helminth affecting human.

2. Despite improvement in living standard children are frequently affected specially in the developing countries. In many communities prevalence may be in excess of 80% [8, 28].

3. Roughly one-quarter of the population are affected.

4. Majority of the patients are asymptomatic.

5. Symptoms develop when worm burden is high.

6. Ascariasis has enormous morbidity and affects many organs in the body but fatalities are usually due to intestinal and pancreatico-biliary ascariasis.

7. Inspite of modernization, ascariasis is regarded as neglected tropical disease.

8. Lozano R et al. in Lancet (December 2012) reported ascariasis caused about 2700 directly attributable death down from 3400 in 1990 [29]. Indirectly attributable death due to malnutrition may be much higher.

9. Health education, improvement of personal hygiene, improvement of sanitation in community, proper disposal of human faeces,providing clean drinking water are all important to help eradication of the disease.

10. Albendazole is the drug of choice for ascariasis with cure rate over 95% and gradual reduction of eggs in the next few weeks in 99.5%

11. Patient with intestinal obstruction and pancreatico biliary complications, a very high index of suspicion is of paramount importance specially in the endemic areas in order to avoid serious complications.

12. No effective vaccine for human trial available till date.

Author details

Narendra Nath Mukhopadhyay
Department of Surgery, Gouri Devi Institute of Medical Sciences, Rajbandh, India

*Address all correspondence to: narendranath.mukherjee@yahoo.com

References

[1] Andrade-junior DR, Karam JA, Wasth MPT, Marca AF, Jukemura J, Machado MCC, et al. Massive infestation by *Ascaris lumbricoides* of the biliary tract: Report of a successfully treated case. Revista do Instituto de Medicina Tropical de São Paulo. 1992;**31**:71-75

[2] Elkins DB, Haswell-Elkins M, Anderson RM. The epidemiology and control of intestinal helminthes in the Pulicat region of Southern India. 1. Study design and pre- and post-treatment observations on *Ascarislumbricoides* infection. Transactions of the Royal Society of Tropical Medicine and Hygiene. 1986;**80**:774-792

[3] Henry FJ, Huttly SRA, Ahmed MU, Alam A. Effect of chemotherapy on helminth reinfection in slums and villages in Bangladesh. The Southeast Asian Journal of Tropical Medicine and Public Health. 1993;**24**:307-312

[4] Fahim SM, Das S, Gazi MA, Mahfuz M, Ahmed T. Association of intestinal pathogens with faecal markers of environmental enteric dysfunction among slum-dwelling children in the first 2 years of life in Bangladesh. Tropical Medicine & International Health. 2018;**23**(11):1242-1250

[5] Darlington CD, Anitha GFS. Ascaridial volvulus: An uncommon cause of ileal perforation. Iranian Journal of Medical Sciences. 2018;**43**(4):432-435

[6] Zakzuk J, Casadiego S, Mercado A, Alvis-Guzman N, Caraballo L. *Ascaris lumbricoides* infection induces both, reduction and increase of asthma symptoms in a rural community. Acta Tropica. 2018;**187**:1-4

[7] Dold C, Holland CV. Ascaris and ascariasis. Microbes and Infection. 2011;**13**(7):632-637

[8] Arfaa F. Selective primary health care: Strategies for control of disease in the developing World. XII. Ascariasis and Trichuriasis. Reviews of Infectious Diseases. 1984;**6**:364-373

[9] Sharma M, Somani P, Prasad R, Jindal S, Pathak A. Biliary ascariasis: Mimicker of biliary stent. VideoGIE. 2017;**2**(7):179-181

[10] Sharma A, Jariwala P, Kaur N. Biliary ascariasis presenting with gangrenous perforation of the gall bladder: Report of a case and brief review of literature. Tropical Doctor. 2018;**48**(3):242-245

[11] Gelpi AP, Mustafa A. Seasonal pneumonitis and eosinophilia. A study of larval ascariasis in Saudi Arabs. The American Journal of Tropical Medicine and Hygiene. 1967;**16**:646-657

[12] Toutai C et al. Uncommon Ascaris induced Eosinophilic Myocarditis simulating acute coronary syndrome without ST segment elevation: A case report. Annals of Medicine and Surgery. 2012;**76**(2022):103522

[13] Lagundoye SB. Disordered small bowel pattern in ascariasis. Tropical and Geographical Medicine. 1972;**24**:226-231

[14] Stephenson LS, Crompton DW, Latham MC, Arnold SE, Jansen AA. Evaluation of a four year project to control *Ascaris* infection in children in two Kenyan villages. Journal of Tropical Pediatrics. 1983;**29**:175-184

[15] Hadidjaja P, Bonang GE, Arifin-Suyardi M, Alisan S, Abidin N, Suhariah- Ismid IS, et al. The effect of intervention methods on nutritional status and cognitive function of primary school children infected with *Ascaris*

lumbricoides. The American Journal of Tropical Medicine and Hygiene. 1998;**59**:791-795

[16] Blumenthal DS, Schultz MG. Incidence of intestinal obstruction in children infected with *Ascaris lumbricoides*. The American Journal of Tropical Medicine and Hygiene. 1975;**24**:801-805

[17] de Silva NR, Guyatt HL, Bundy DA. Morbidity and mortality due to *Ascaris*-induced intestinal obstruction. Transactions of The Royal Society of Tropical Medicine and Hygiene. 1997;**91**:31-36

[18] Villamizar E, Mendez M, Bonilla E, Varon H, Onatra de S. *Ascaris lumbricoides* infestation as a cause of intestinal obstruction in children: Experience with 87 cases. Journal of Pediatric Surgery. 1996;**31**:201-205

[19] Mukhopadhyay NN, Mukherjee P, Ali SKS, et al. *Ascaris lumbricoides* Causing Duodeno-ureteric Fistula. The Indian Journal of Surgery. 2022. DOI: 10.1007/s12262-022-03349-9

[20] Pawlowski ZS, Arfaa F. Ascariasis. In: Warren KS, Mahmoud AAF, editors. Tropical and Geographical Medicine. New York: McGraw-Hill Book Company; 1985. pp. 347-358

[21] Xianmin Z, Weidong P, Crompton DWT, Jaingqin X. Treatment of biliary ascariasis in China. Transactions of the Royal Society of Tropical Medicine and Hygiene. 1999;**93**:561-564

[22] Asrat T, Rogers N. Acute pancreatitis caused by biliary *Ascaris* in pregnancy. Journal of Perinatology. 1985;**15**:326-332

[23] Mascarini-Serra L. Prevention of soil-transmitted Helminth infection. Journal of Global Infectious Diseases. 2011;**3**(2):175-182. DOI: 10.4103/0974-777X.81696

[24] WHO. Preventive Chemotherapy in Human Helminthiasis: Coordinated Use of Anthelminthic Drugs in Control Interventions : A Manual for Health Professionals and Programme Managers (PDF). 2006. WHO Press, World Health Organization, Geneva, Switzerland. pp. 1-61. ISBN 978-9241547109. Archived (PDF) from the original on 2013-02-28

[25] Keiser J, Utzinger J. The drugs we have and the drugs we need against major helminth infections. Advances in Parasitology. 2010;**73**:197-230

[26] Gazzinelli-Guimarães A, Gazzinelli-Guimarães P, Weatherhead J. A historical and systematic overview of Ascaris vaccine development. Parasitology. 2021;**148**(14):1795-1805. DOI: 10.1017/S0031182021001347

[27] Ghosh G, Shah S, Maltz C. Ascariasis diagnosed by wireless capsule endoscopy. Clinical Gastroenterology and Hepatology. 2018;**16**(6):A23

[28] Croll NA, Anderson RM, Gyorkos TW, Chadiran E. The population biology and control of *Ascaris lumbricoides* in a rural community in Iran. Transactions of the Royal Society of Tropical Medicine and Hygiene. 1982;**76**:187-197

[29] Lozano R, Naghavi M, Foreman K, Lim S, Shibuya K, Aboyans V, et al. Global and regional mortality from 235 causes of death for 20 age groups in 1990 and 2010: A systematic analysis for the Global Burden of Disease Study 2010. Lancet. 2012;**380**(9859):2095-2128. DOI: 10.1016/S0140-6736(12)61728-0 hdl: 10536/DRO/DU:30050819

Chapter 5

Trichuris: A Critical Review

Parvaiz Yousuf, Semran Parvaiz, Shahid Razzak and Nisheet Zehbi

Abstract

Trichuris (whipworms) is a type of roundworm that is responsible for trichuriasis in human beings. Globally, 600–800 million people are infected by this helminthic worm per year. *Trichuris* is more prevalent in some tropical and sub-tropical areas such as East Asia, China, Sub-Saharan Africa, and the Americas. These parasitic nematodes affect the small intestines of mammals, causing a great deal of discomfort. Their life cycle is completed in two stages; mammals and the external environment. The zoonotic transmission of the disease is responsible for huge infections and deaths around the world. In recent times, researchers have gained a lot of understanding about the genetics and parasitology of *Trichuris*. In this chapter, we will discuss the origin, phylogeny, life cycle, diagnosis, and zoonotic transmission of the parasite. At the same time, the chapter discusses the genomics of the parasite and the future directions that can help us contain this parasitic nematode.

Keywords: Trichuris, trichuriasis, whipworms, *Trichuris trichiura*, parasitology

1. Introduction

Soilborne helminths affect roughly a quarter of the world's population or 1.5 billion people. Especially prevalent in East Asia, sub-Saharan Africa, the Americas, and China, soilborne helminthiasis is found across the tropics and sub-tropics. More than 568 million school-aged children and 267 million preschoolers need treatment and prevention measures because they reside in locations with high rates of these parasites' spread. Humans are most commonly infected with *Ascaris lumbricoides* (roundworm), *Trichuris trichiura* (whipworm), *Necator americanus*, and *Ancylostoma duodenale*, all of which are soil-dwelling helminths (hookworms) [1]. The nematode parasite *Trichuris trichiura* is responsible for causing trichuriasis, a condition that is often overlooked despite its pathogenicity. Trichuriasis, caused by T. *trichiura*, is the second most prevalent helminth infection in humans and is found in every region of the world. The incidence rate is greater in areas with tropical climates where proper sanitary facilities are lacking. The greatest parasite burden and the most noticeable symptoms are seen in children, who account for 30–80% of cases [2]. This parasite is spread through the oral consumption of its embryonic eggs. New hosts can contract the disease from infected hands, food, soil, or water. These then develop into L1 larvae, which are passed out of the body after hatching in the intestine. The larvae eat their way through the large intestine's epithelial lining and mature into adults.

The females lay their unfertilized eggs into the environment after mating, and the eggs once again enter the environment via the excrement of their hosts. To this day, T. *trichiura* has remained the species of choice for describing whipworms found in primates [3–5]; *Trichuris suis* refers to those found in domestic pigs and wild boars [6, 7]. The phenotypic flexibility of the organisms, variation generated by the host, a lack of morphological traits, and the overlapping of morphological characteristics across closely related species of *Trichuris* make accurate identification of one species from another a formidable challenge [8–11]. Because of their molecular differences but comparable morphologies, T. *trichiura* and T. *suis* have been the focus of numerous *Trichuris*-related investigations [7, 12–14].

Trichuris is a protozoan parasite that has been found in humans and nonhuman primates (NHP), although the genetic and evolutionary ties between the two are unclear. Whether or not *Trichuris* species are shared by humans and NHP has been the subject of some recent publications. Due to its widespread distribution and ability to infect a wide variety of hosts, the genus *Trichuris* is an excellent candidate for hiding cryptic species [15]. Recent research has shown that more than one taxon of T. *trichiura* is able to infect humans and other primates, including captive animals, suggesting that this species is more complicated than previously thought [16, 17]. *Trichuris rhinopiptheroxella*, discovered in the golden snub-nosed monkey (*Rhinopithecus roxellana*), *Trichuris colobae* from *Colobus guereza kikuyuensis*, and *Trichuris ursinus* from *Papio ursinus* have all been reported based on morpho-biometric and molecular data [18–20]. As a result of these findings, T. *trichiura* is not the only whipworm discovered in primates. The systematics of the genus *Trichuris* currently have substantial gaps. This is due to two major factors: i) a lack of comparative morpho-biometric data obtained through the application of multiple parameters and statistical tests to the taxonomic study of these species, and (ii) a scarcity of published research on the genetics of the various *Trichuris* species in humans, NHP, and pigs. Researchers have yet to determine the degree of divergence between the several genetic lineages that appear to exist in *Trichuris* species that parasitize these hosts. We shall try to understand the morphological and biometric properties of T. *trichiura* isolated from people in this chapter. Moreover, molecular data (mitochondrial and nuclear markers) are used to describe the molecular phylogenetic relationships between these populations. Furthermore, we shall attempt to comprehend the origin, life cycle, taxonomy, transmission, and resistance of the *Trichuris* spp.

2. The origin of the species

Whipworms are parasitic nematodes that inhabit the intestines of mammals. Due to their distinctive form, which comprises of a long, thin front end (the stichosome) that embeds in the intestinal epithelial cells of its host, and a bulbous rear end, all whipworm species share the generic name *Trichuris*, meaning "hair tail." In 1761, Roederer gave the parasite the name *Trichuris* after mistaking its head for its tail. There are more than seventy different species of *Trichuris*, and a number of these parasites have significant roles in medicine, veterinary science, and fundamental research. The human whipworm is an example of a parasite that co-evolved with humans, earning it the moniker "heirloom parasite." Due to the discovery of whipworm eggs in both Old and New World archeological sites, evidence of a link between the whipworm and prehistoric man dates back more than 6000 years [21]. Mice infected with *Trichuris* were first studied by parasitologists curious about the

Year	Researcher	Findings	Ref.
1761	Roederer et al.	He gave the parasite the name *Trichuris* after mistaking its head for its tail	[21]
1858	Davaine et al.	Described the process of embryonation in *Trichuris Spp*	[23]
1954	Fahmy et al.	Defined the environmental requirements for the first stage of larval development within the egg	[22]
1989	Panesar et al.	Defined the complete sequence of larval molts from L1 through L4 to adult	[24]
2008	Araujo et al.	Discovery of whipworm eggs in both Old and New World archeological sites	[21]

Table 1.
The people involved in the identification of Trichirus trichiura.

parasite, its life cycle, and parasite biology. Eventually, parasite immunologists took use of T. *muris* infections in laboratory mice to investigate host–parasite interactions immunologically, with the ultimate goal of developing vaccines to increase resistance to infection. The value of intestinal worm infections as tools for testing the immune system and addressing fundamental immunological topics has also been recognized by immunologists who study more advanced immunological concerns. Parasite biology and the roles that parasite chemicals play in disease have received fresh attention in recent years. This renaissance is due to the desire to find parasite immunomodulatory chemicals that may have therapeutic applications for inflammatory diseases of the developed world and the scarcity of lead antigens for use in vaccines. From a parasitological perspective, characterizing the full life cycle of the *Trichuris* parasite required a long time (**Table 1**).

Davaine initially described the process of embryonation in *Trichuris* spp. Eggs and Fahmy defined the environmental requirements for the first stage of larval development within the egg [22, 23]. Recently, it was discovered by accident that slightly acidic water hinders embryonation and results in failure in egg cultures in laboratories throughout the world that maintain the *Trichuris* life cycle. These discoveries are still relevant today because of this thing. Before Fahmy outlined a more accurate direct life cycle involving two larval molts and fecund adult parasites emerging around day 34, there were early misconceptions regarding the life cycle, including descriptions of migratory phases [22]. The complete sequence of larval molts from L1 through L4 to adult was not determined until the 1980s [24].

2.1 Taxonomy and Phylogenetics

Trichuris is a genus of the worm family Enoplea, in the suborder Trichinellida, together with *Trichinella spiralis*. There are 16 recognized species of *Trichuris*, which live in a wide variety of mammalian hosts, according to the NCBI Taxonomy Browser. Although *Trichuris suis* in pigs is the closest relative of *Trichuris trichiura*, it is still unclear whether *Trichuris* in dogs and rodents (*Trichuris vulpis*, *Trichuris arvicolae*, *Trichuris muris*) or ruminants (*Trichuris ovis, Trichuris discolor, Trichuris skrjabini*) diverged before or after *Trichuris trichiura* [25–28]. *Trichuris trichiura* is the scientific name for human whipworms. At the same time, it was previously considered that just one species of whipworm infected humans, but recent articles have begun to study the potential that numerous species exist in the human population.

Because of its extensive distribution and ability to infect a wide variety of host species, the *Trichuris* genus is a likely candidate for cryptic species, which are parasites that cannot be identified as species by standard approaches such as morphological research (**Figure 1**) [29]. For a more in-depth look at the taxonomic relationship between *Trichuris* parasites in humans and NHP, as well as the potential for cross-species transmission, *Trichuris* parasites were sampled from a wide range of wild and captive NHP host species and then sequenced their nuclear and mitochondrial markers. Internal transcribed spacer (ITS) sequences were compared between *Trichuris* from baboons in the wild on the Cape Peninsula of South Africa and *Trichuris* from humans and pigs [30]. *Trichuris* in humans was found to be divided into two clades (DG and CP-COB), both of which were also found in baboons. Full mitochondrial DNA (mtDNA) genome study of worms from humans in China and Uganda, as well as baboons in the United States and Denmark, produced comparable results [31]. Genetic divergence between these worms reached as high as 20%, suggesting that *Trichuris* in humans consists of multiple species and that parasite transmission between humans and baboons is possible. *Trichuris* samples collected from baboons in captivity in Denmark and the United States were revealed, through sequence analysis of the conserved beta-tubulin gene, to be members of the same evolutionary group as human *Trichuris* samples from Uganda [32]. An examination of *Trichuris* samples from humans and a variety of NHP species in and around Kibale National Park in Uganda revealed a similar separation of primate *Trichuris* into separate clades as documented by Ravasi *et al.* [33].

The clade CP-GOB was further separated into two groups, one with *Trichuris* from colobus and yellow-cheeked gibbon and the other with *Trichuris* from eight primate host species, including humans [33]. *Trichuris* mitochondrial and nuclear marker sequencing on the critically endangered Francois' leaf monkey indicated the possibility of a new *Trichuris* species. A recent in-depth study has added new, never-before-seen evidence to the phylogeny given by Callejon *et al.* [27, 34, 35]. The authors

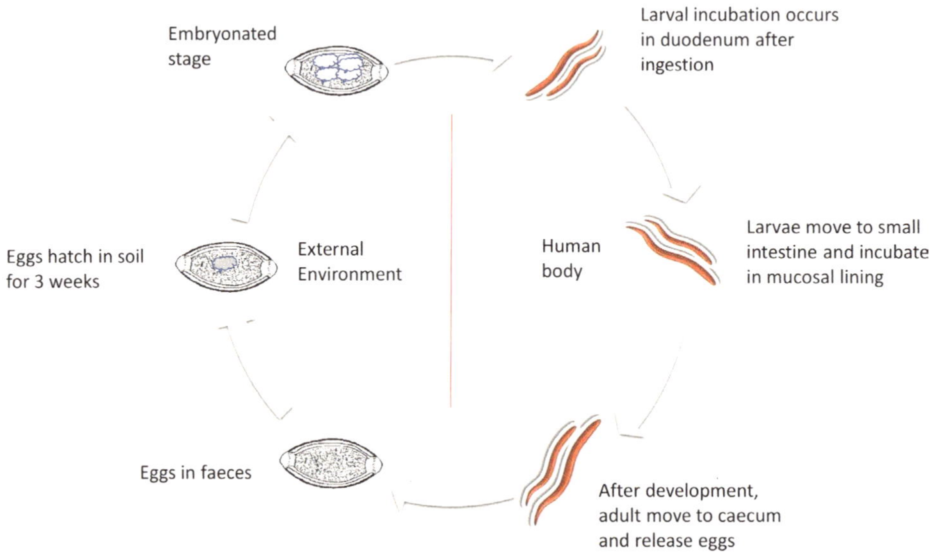

Figure 1.
Life cycle of Trichuris.

proposed that there are two subclades within clade 2 (baboon and human *Trichuris* and macaque *Trichuris*), and at least two subclades within clade 1 (*Trichuris* from a range of primate species including humans) and *SUIS* (*Trichuris* from pigs and occasionally humans), with *Trichuris* from black-and-white colobus and gibbons falling into subclade CA or a separate grouping depending on the phylog *Trichuris colobae*, a new *Trichuris* species based on morphological criteria, was recently reported from black and white colobuses [36]. Similar to the work of Cavallero *et al.*, this study determined that François' leaf-monkey *Trichuris* belongs to a distinct subclade based on its ITS sequences. It's probable that the whipworms that plague people are actually different species of the nematode parasite *Trichuris*, some of which are also seen in ungulates [27, 31].

Because current studies have been limited by a small number of human samples from only a few sites, and because different researchers have used different genetic markers, it is possible that more species or subspecies will be identified in the future. Recently, the rrnL gene of the mtDNA of *Trichuris* from persons in China (n = 7) and Ecuador (n = 15) was sequenced and compared genetically [37]. Worms from the same geographical location tended to cluster together, showing a phylogeographic pattern; nonetheless, it is unclear whether these worms are distinct subspecies. Further investigation of the taxonomic relationship between worms necessitates the collection of more worm samples from humans and NHPs all over the world, as well as the use of various genetic markers.

The ITS region has been the primary focus of previous studies; however, because of its high repetition content, even alignments of closely related worm sequences would include gaps. This complicates worm phylogenetic studies. Hence it's recommended that additional genetic markers, including mitochondrial DNA genes, be used [27, 30, 33, 35, 38, 39].

3. Life cycle, development, and diagnosis

T. *trichiura* eggs have a unique barrel shape and measure 50–54 lm in length and 22 lm in breadth when oviposited in the large intestine. Before hatching into infectious larvae, the eggs must spend around 3 weeks in the soil at the proper temperature and humidity. As a result, the optimal circumstances are shady, warm, and wet soil. Eggs will not grow in direct sunlight and will perish if the temperature falls below 9 degrees Celsius or rises beyond 52 degrees Celsius. It is unknown what happens to the larvae in the first 5–10 days after they are consumed by humans (**Figure 2**). The larvae first enter the duodenum, where they stay for about a week before reentering the intestinal lumen and moving to the caecum, where they burrow into the mucosal surface via their anterior ends, according to most parasitology textbooks. However, there are contradictory findings from animal research and no human studies of the duodenal phase [40]. After hatching in the duodenum, T. *vulpis* larvae have been shown to develop in the caecum, piercing the mucosal epithelium and re-emerging into the lumen 8–10 days later. The major evidence for this approach comes from serial necropsies of diseased dogs performed for up to 10 days [41]. A dose of this magnitude could have stimulated migration to abnormal locations. Due to insufficient histological monitoring of the caecal mucosa over the course of 10 days, it is possible that all larvae identified there first entered the mucosa.

There needs to be more investigation into whether or not the duodenum phase of *Trichuris* spp. is an experimental artifact or an actual stage in the life cycle.

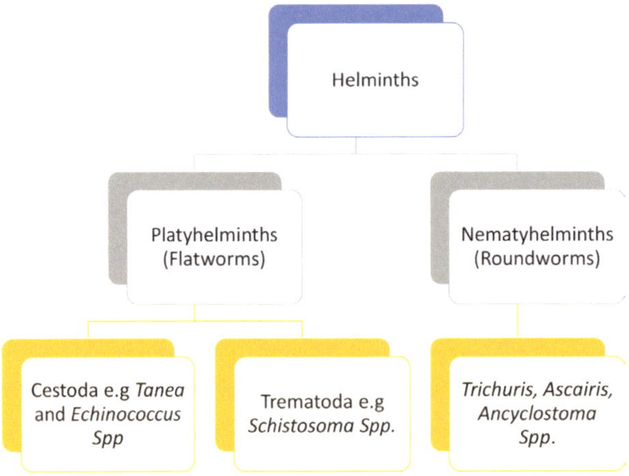

Figure 2.
The classification of Trichuris.

Investigations using pigs infected with physiological doses of T. *suis* eggs may serve as the most accurate model for human infection and provide valuable background for future studies on humans. Adult T. *trichiura* appears 30–90 days after infection, and after mating, the females start laying eggs. All researchers agree that it is common to find adult worms in the epithelium lining the caecum and colon. In severe infections, worms may also be found in other parts of the gastrointestinal tract, including the appendix, rectum, and distal ileum. Like a whip, an adult worm's body is divided between a thicker, more rounded section at the back (the handle) and a thinner, more tapered section up front (the lash). The length of an adult worm is between 3 and 5 centimeters, with females being somewhat longer. Laboratory investigations of T. *muris* have revealed that the worm's anterior segment is ensconced in a syncytium (or mass of cytoplasm) generated from enterocytes [42]. It appears that the parasite is using its anterior stylet to burrow inside this tube.

Cytolytic enzymes are secreted from the mouth and the bacillary band on the ventral cuticle. This thicker rear end stretches into the caecal lumen, making mating and oviposition much easier. If the worms are able to penetrate the basement membranes of the enterocytes, they will be able to ingest not only the syncytium but also the erythrocytes, leucocytes, mucosaluids, and cells that are present in the gastrointestinal tract [43]. The Kato-Katz thick smear is the gold standard for this purpose; it is used in field surveys to identify hookworm and *A. lumbricoides* and to assess the degree of infection in eggs per gramme of feces (EPG) [44]. Some hospital-based researchers have used anoscopy to see adult worms in the rectum to diagnose severe trichuriasis, as the worm population extends all the way down to the lower colon in cases of severe trichuriasis [45]. In extreme cases, the worm population can extend as far down the lower colon as the rectum. Hence some hospital-based researchers have used anoscopy to detect adult worms in the rectum to diagnose severe trichuriasis [46]. A total of 187 people of varying ages in a St. Lucian village and 120 schoolchildren in the Tanga region of Tanzania were used for the study. Anti-T. *trichiura* salivary IgG responses were higher in children with active *Trichuris* infection compared to children without infection, and the age associations of parasite-specific salivary IgG antibodies mirrored those of infection severity in the general population. This method may be used as a community-wide gauge of transmission ferocity; however, its widespread adoption will depend in part on its suitability for in-house use and per-case cost.

3.1 Zoonotic transmission

Many people believe that *Trichuris trichiura* is the sole causative agent of human trichuriasis; however, there is evidence of infection with additional *Trichuris* species in humans and of zoonotic transmission of *Trichuris* parasites. The dog- and wolf-infecting parasite *Trichuris vulpis* has been hypothesized to be transmitted to humans due to the identification of its unusually large eggs in human feces [47].

Trichuris trichiura eggs can be little or large, and females may deposit eggs that are similar in size to *Trichuris vulpis* eggs [47, 48]. Eleven percent of *Trichuris*-positive kids in Thailand were found to have *Trichuris vulpis* eggs in their poop when tested using molecular markers, highlighting the parasite's zoonotic potential in the area [49]. Because *Trichuris suis* is more closely related to *Trichuris trichiura*, it is assumed that this parasite, which naturally infects pigs and can cause significant economic losses in pig production, is more likely to be transmitted to humans. Morphological analysis, however, cannot tell *Trichuris trichiura* eggs, larvae, and adults from *Trichuris suis* [25]. This means that traditional parasitological methods are useless for detecting probable cases of host–host cross-transmission. Recently, there have been endeavors to use genetic approaches to better understand *Trichuris suis*'s zoonotic potential. Three out of a total of 29 worms collected from people in Uganda who shared their environment with pigs were positive for *Trichuris suis*, as reported by Nissen *et al*. [14]. They sequenced the beta-tubulin gene and analyzed the ITS-2 region using PCR-RFLP. Nuclear and mitochondrial markers were not able to detect *Trichuris suis* in either people or pigs in rural Ecuador [50]. This genetic exchange between *Trichuris trichiura* and *Trichuris suis* was detected in two pig *Trichuris* samples, which had a Bheterozygous-type PCR-RFLP pattern. However, the sample size (n = 16) was too small to draw any firm conclusions on the possibility of cross-species transmission based on sequencing of the ITS region and the rrnL gene of *Trichuris* from pigs and humans in China [26, 51]. To assess the scope and significance of *Trichuris* transmission between domestic animals and humans, more sympatric sampling of *Trichuris* from humans, dogs, or pigs in various geographic locations, together with DNA analysis, is recommended and required. Several wild NHP species, including colobus monkeys, macaques, baboons, and chimps, have tested positive for *Trichuris* infections [27–29]. The aforementioned molecular studies suggest that certain *Trichuris* species are restricted to certain NHPs, while other *Trichuris* species are genetically identical to humans and could therefore spread across the two groups. This has crucial consequences for human health and wildlife conservation when NHPs and people coexist, as is increasingly the case as humans encroach onto pristine ecosystems and NHPs gain access to gardens and farms in search of food.

3.2 Anthelmintic resistance

By 2020, the World Health Organization (WHO) hopes to provide preventative chemotherapy to 75 percent of all preschool and school-age children who are at risk. This goal can be met by regularly distributing benzimidazole anthelminthic medicines to school-aged children, such as single-dose albendazole or mebendazole (**Table 2**) [30, 31, 52]. Treatment of *Trichuris* with a single dosage of albendazole or

Treatment	Mechanism of action	Egg reduction rate (%age)	Cure rate (%age)
Albendazole	β- Tubulin binding	64.3	32.1
Mebendazole	β- Tubulin binding	80.7	44.4
Pyrantel pamoate	L- subtype nAChR agonist	62.3	28.5
Levamisole	L- subtype nAChR agonist	41.8	23.4
Albendazole–ivermectin	N/A	95.5	60.0

Table 2.
The drugs used in the treatment and their mechanism of action [53].

mebendazole has a low success rate (between 30 and 70 percent) [53]. Some people are worried about the rise of drug resistance [32, 33, 54, 55]. Due to their widespread usage, anthelmintics have bred resistance in nematodes of veterinary importance, including those that cause gastrointestinal parasitism in ruminants and horses [34–37]. A single nucleotide polymorphism (SNP) in the parasite beta-tubulin gene that causes phenylalanine to be substituted by tyrosine at codon 200 is a common source of benzimidazole drug resistance [38]. Resistance is sometimes also associated with nonsynonymous SNPs at codons 167 and 198 [39, 56]. An early investigation of sequence variation in the beta-tubulin gene of 72 *Trichuris trichiura* isolates from seven countries identified no alterations linked with benzimidazole resistance [57]. It was projected that antihelmintic resistance would arise more slowly in *Trichuris trichiura* than in trichostrongyles from domesticated animals due to its lower genetic diversity and smaller population size. Recently, pyrosequencing techniques have been developed to detect nonsynonymous SNPs at codons 167, 198, and 200 in *Trichuris trichiura* and other soil-transmitted helminths [58, 59]. These SNPs are present naturally in whipworm populations since 2.6% of *Trichuris* samples from Kenyan newborns who were assumed to have not had benzimidazole treatment were homozygous for the resistance mutation at codon 200. Furthermore, the codon 200 mutation associated with resistance was present in five out of eight *Trichuris trichiura* egg pools collected from children treated with a single dose of albendazole [58].

In *Trichuris trichiura* samples from Kenya and Haiti that were collected before and after treatment with albendazole, there was a significant increase in the homozygous resistance genotype at codon 200 of beta-tubulin, and this was associated with low rates of egg reduction [59]. It was also discovered that *Trichuris* from Panama had polymorphisms at codons 198 and 167. By contrast, Hansen *et al.* detected no SNPs in *Trichuris* from captive baboons, Ugandan people, wild animals, and domestic animals at beta-tubulin codons 167, 198, or 200 [60, 61]. However, 41 percent of human *Trichuris* samples were collected via mebendazole chemoexpulsion, which may explain why no resistance SNPs were detected. Because only worms without the resistance marker are ejected, it stands to reason that resistance markers are less common when using DNA retrieved from evicted worms. The beta-tubulin genotypes of eggs found in feces can be used to learn more about the resistant and non-resistant mother worms that lay them. More research is needed to prove that benzimidazole treatment increases the frequency of these mutations and that these SNPs are responsible for the reduced efficacy of albendazole and mebendazole in treating human trichuriasis, but existing data show that SNPs in the beta-tubulin gene are present in whipworms and are associated with anthelmintic resistance in other nematodes. The fact that the adult form of *Trichuris trichiura* dwells in the large intestine may explain why anthelmintics are ineffective, but it is far from the only explanation. The *Trichuris trichiura* worm's front segment is embedded in the intestinal mucosa, which may contribute to poor treatment outcomes. As a result, even though the anthelmintic momentarily paralyzes the worms, the worms remain attached to the host and can recover if the therapy is stopped. *Trichuris* may be able to excrete the medication via P-glycoprotein-mediated transport [62], despite the fact that the drug is thought to enter the worms by passive diffusion [63].

3.3 Ancient DNA

Evidence of human *Trichuris* infection dating back thousands of years have been discovered through paleoparasitological studies, even in regions where the parasite is now uncommon, such as Europe and North America. Eggs of the parasitic worm *Trichuris* have been found in a variety of artifacts from the ancient world, including human feces, feces from other animals, coprolites, and latrines [64, 65]. Paleoparasitological research has traditionally relied on morphological analyses of parasite eggs, which only allow for genus-level identification. When working with old samples, the fundamental problem is the degradation of DNA into minute bits that are not amplifiable using traditional PCR. Recent advances in DNA extraction technology, as well as the amplification and sequencing of small species-specific amplicons, have enabled the identification of ancient DNA from parasite eggs [66, 67]. To this end, longer sequences homologous to *Trichuris trichiura* have been reconstructed from archeological finds in Denmark (1030 AD) and Korea (1755 AD) by focusing on tiny overlapping portions of *Trichuris* 18S SSUrRNA [67]. As science and technology advance, it may be possible to obtain more in-depth genomic insights from ancient parasites, shining a light on their distributions and migration patterns throughout history.

3.4 Genomics and transcriptomics

The advancement of high-throughput genomic and transcriptomic technologies has ushered in a new era in which a wholly novel technique can give extraordinary insights into parasite molecular biology [68]. The recent publication of the genomes of *Trichuris trichiura*, *Trichuris muris*, and *Trichuris suis* marks a major milestone in *Trichuris* studies [69]. Furthermore, transcriptome analysis confirmed the genomes of *Trichuris suis* and *Trichuris muris*, providing a thorough understanding of the chemicals and genes expressed by these parasites during invasion, survival, and interaction with their hosts. *Trichuris trichiura* has a smaller genome (75.2 MBin) and fewer genes (9650) than *Trichuris suis* (male: 83.6 MB; female: 87.2 MB; 14,781 genes) and *Trichuris muris* (85.0 MB; 11,004 genes), although many of these genes are preserved [69]. There are two sets of autosomes and one set of X and Y sex chromosomes in *Trichuris muris* (2n = 6), and it appears that *Trichuris trichiura* has the same karyotype. Numerous genes in the genomes have been predicted to play a role in parasite–host interactions and immuno-regulation (or immunological modulation) of the infected host.

There are 618 predicted excretory-secretory proteins in *Trichuris suis*, and while secretory proteins only make up about 4% of the gene set, they are responsible for 10% of the genes that are actually transcribed [70]. Furthermore, both *Trichuris muris* and *Trichuris suis* overexpressed proteases and protease inhibitors, showing that these molecules play an important role in host-tissue disintegration and in regulating protein activities relevant to immunomodulation [70]. Genome-guided drug development [71] uses information from genomes and transcriptomes to identify potential therapeutic compounds with high parasite specificity. Hundreds of proteins were identified as potential pharmacological targets for *Trichuris suis* and *Trichuris trichiura*. However, Foth *et al.* narrowed the list down to 29 top protein choices that were homologs to targets for currently available drugs [69]. Jex *et al.* investigated the significance of short non-coding RNAs in gene regulation, and their central role as gene regulators suggests that these RNA species could be novel therapeutic targets [70, 72].

4. Future research directions

Because of decreasing assay costs and simpler implementation of B-omic-based techniques, including genomic, transcriptomic, epigenomic, and proteomic research, novel insights into *Trichuris* biology are predicted in the future years. Advances have paved the path for population-level comparative investigations of whole genome sequencing [73], which have the potential to completely alter *Trichuris* phylogenetic and evolutionary investigations. This will lead to a much more precise understanding of distribution patterns and the discovery of new subspecies and hybridization occurrences between existing species. Since anthelmintic therapies are generally ineffective, the lack of readily available worms will continue to be a significant barrier to genetic research on *Trichuris*. The proteome of the non-embryonated eggs of *T. trichiura* as a unique source of data on prospective targets for immunodiagnostics and immunomodulators from a neglected tropical disease was investigated by Cruz *et al.* and a list of *T. trichiura* non-embryonated egg proteins (proteome and antigenic profile) was provided which can be used in future research into the pathophysiology and immunobiology of human trichuriasis, as well as the management of disorders of the human intestinal immune system [74]. A number of potential new drugs have been found thanks to the whole-genome sequencing of *Trichuris trichiura*, which may make worm collection less of a hassle in the future [69]. However, as the necessary input sample for comparative studies decreases fast, it is expected that widely available feces samples containing *Trichuris* eggs will become crucial to large-scale studies. Single cells have yielded whole genome sequences and even transcriptomes [75], which allows similar experiments on embryonated eggs containing hundreds of cells could be possible in the near future. Micromanipulation, which has allowed researchers to pick individual helminth eggs for subsequent PCR-based amplification, could be a first step [76]. While there does appear to be a pattern of infection with distinct *Trichuris* species infecting distinct host species, there are still a number of questions that require answering. To what extent can pathology, epidemiology, and drug susceptibility vary across *Trichuris* spp. that infect humans, and can numerous *Trichuris* spp. be found in the same area? In what ways, if any, do NHPs naturally transmit *Trichuris* to humans? Can *Trichuris* from one clade infect hosts from another clade, or are the various *Trichuris* species in primates host specific? These mysteries have only recently begun to be unveiled, and additional research is needed that employs multiple genetic marker manufacturers to analyze *Trichuris* samples from people and NHPs from sympatric regions and around the world. This will shed light on the pathways through which parasites are transmitted between these monkeys, paving the way for more effective measures of control and prevention to be put in place.

Another important topic for future study is the dissection of host–parasite interactions; this is a goal shared by the "50 Helminth Genomes project" and the

"959 Nematode Genomes" initiative [77]. These genomes will shed new light on the molecular biology and evolutionary history of helminth parasites, a field that has been largely overlooked until now. The host stimulus-induced hatching of *Trichuris* eggs during transit through the small intestine is a poorly understood mechanism in *Trichuris* development. *Trichuris suis* eggs require a different set of stimuli for hatching than *Trichuris muris* eggs do, demonstrating the extreme host–parasite specificity of this phenomenon [78]. Genome and transcriptome data from the protozoan parasites *Trichuris suis* and *Trichuris muris* have improved our understanding of other mechanisms, such as the parasites' ability to establish themselves in the host and to avoid the host immune system [69, 70]. Unpublished transcriptome data from *Trichuris trichiura* will also definitely contribute new insights. Exosomes are tiny microvesicles (about 30–100 nm in size) that are employed for intercellular communication in complex organisms. Interesting new research shows that parasites also make and discharge exosomes containing microRNA that can be absorbed by host cells. Intriguingly, exosomes released by the gastrointestinal worm *Heligmosomoides polygyrus* have been found to inhibit type 2 innate response in mice and activate certain immune genes in vitro [79]. Similarly, it was demonstrated that *Trichuris suis*, like other protozoa, secretes vesicles of exosome size that contain RNA, although the function of these vesicles is still a mystery [80]. Future research should define the contents of these exosomes and investigate their role in the host–parasite interaction, such as whether *Trichuris* uses exosomes to manipulate the host's immune response in order to decrease inflammation and optimize its survival. Genotyping of ancient *Trichuris* eggs is anticipated to become more common in paleoparasitology. Because *Trichuris* spp. has a limited host range, genotyping a specific egg discovery has been suggested as a suitable approach to determine the host of origin, which gives paleoparasitologists a tool for studying prehistoric host–parasite interactions. In addition, investigations of historical migration patterns can benefit greatly from the information provided by genotyping *Trichuris* eggs. The question of how *Trichuris trichiura* got to the Americas is still up for grabs. The problem, however, is that *Trichuris trichiura*, like other STH infections, probably cannot be maintained in Arctic conditions, which is exactly what the human journey through the Beringian Land Bridge into the Americas would have required [81]. Point-of-care molecular diagnostics for human trichuriasis are on the horizon, and they may be used in tandem with other STH illnesses. It is critical that testing can be carried out in low-resource and low-cost situations common in developing countries. Loop-mediated isothermal amplification (LAMP) and its derivatives have been found to be a promising technology in early research. *Strongyloides stercoralis* [82] and Opisthorchis viverrine [83]. DNA has been detected using LAMP after being isolated from human feces samples. The current greatest challenge is sample preparation and how it connects to DNA extraction and detection. This has been done in one device for testing gastroenteric infections, but not for any STHs as of yet [84]. The zoonotic potential of *Trichuris* spp. might be addressed, and the degree and species of human infection revealed through widespread point-of-care testing of stool samples for STHs using molecular-based approaches.

5. Conclusion

In recent years, scientists have increased their knowledge of the genetics of trichuriasis and the parasite *Trichuris*. Their genomes have been made public for *Trichuris trichiura*, *Trichuris suis*, and *Trichuris muris*. Important potential mechanisms of host–parasite interaction and immunomodulation, as well as new treatment targets, have been found in this research. In research on human *Trichuris* trichuira isolates, beta-tubulin gene variants associated with resistance in veterinary-important nematodes have been found infrequently. Recent advances have been made in the phylogeny of *Trichuris*. Infections with *Trichuris* appear to take different forms depending on the host. Infections with *Trichuris trichiura* in nonhuman primates, *Trichuris suis* in pigs, and *Trichuris vulpis* in dogs have all been linked to zoonotic transmission. Future research should concentrate on several genetic marker studies of *Trichuris* gathered from humans, nonhuman primates, pigs, and dogs in sympatric and geographical areas in order to understand more about parasite transmission between host species. The development of sensitive molecular diagnostics that can be employed at the point of care will be supported by new technologies for monitoring the spread of anthelmintic resistance. Any advancement in these domains will be incredibly beneficial for preventing and treating this parasitic sickness.

Conflict of interest

The author(s) declare no conflict of interest.

Author details

Parvaiz Yousuf*, Semran Parvaiz, Shahid Razzak and Nisheet Zehbi
Department of Zoology, Central University of Kashmir, Ganderbal, J&K, India

*Address all correspondence to: saleemparvaiz444@gmail.com

References

[1] World Health Organization. Soil-Transmitted Helminth Infections. 2020. Available from: https://www.who.int/es/news-room/fact-sheets/detail/soil-transmitted-helminth-infections

[2] McDowell MA, Rafati S, editors. Neglected Tropical Diseases-Middle East and North Africa. Vienna: Springer; 2014. DOI: 10.1007/978-3-7091-1613-5

[3] Ravasi DF, O'Riain MJ, Davids F, Illing N. Phylogenetic evidence that two distinct *Trichuris genotypes* infect both humans and nonhuman primates. 7(8):e44187. DOI: 10.1371/journal.pone.0044187

[4] Ghai RR, Chapman CA, Omeja PA, Davies TJ, Goldberg TL. Nodule worm infection in humans and wild primates in Uganda: Cryptic species in a newly identified region of human transmission. PLoS neglected tropical diseases. 2014;**8**(1):e2641

[5] Betson M, Søe MJ, Nejsum P. Human trichuriasis: Whipworm genetics, phylogeny, transmission, and future research directions. Current Tropical Medicine Reports. 2015;**2**(4):209-217

[6] Ooi HK, Tenora F, Itoh K, Kamiya M. Comparative study of *Trichuris trichiura* from nonhuman primates and from man, and their difference with T. *suis*. Journal of Veterinary Medical Science. 1993;**55**(3):363-366

[7] Cutillas C, Callejon R, De Rojas M, Tewes B, Ubeda JM, Ariza C, et al. *Trichuris suis* and *Trichuris trichiura* are different nematode species. Acta tropica. 2009;**111**(3):299-307

[8] Knight RA. Morphological differences in *Trichuris* ovis are associated with different host species. The Journal of Parasitology (USA). 1984;**70**(5):842-843

[9] Špakulová M. Discriminant analysis as a method for the numerical evaluation of taxonomic characters in male trichurid nematodes. Systematic Parasitology. 1994;**29**(2):113-119

[10] Robles MD, Navone GT. Redescription of *Trichuris* laevitestis (Nematoda: trichuridae) from Akodon azarae and Scapteromys aquaticus (sigmodontinae: Cricetidae) in Buenos Aires province, Argentina. Journal of Parasitology. 2006;**92**(5):1053-1057

[11] Robles MD. New species of *Trichuris* (Nematoda: Trichuridae) from Akodon montensis Thomas, 1913, of the Paranaense forest in Argentina. The Journal of parasitology. 2011;**97**(2):319-327

[12] Liu GH, Gasser RB, Su A, Nejsum P, Peng L, Lin RQ, et al. Clear genetic distinctiveness between human-and pig-derived *Trichuris* based on analyses of mitochondrial datasets. PLoS Neglected Tropical Diseases. 2012;**6**(2):e1539

[13] Liu GH, Zhou W, Nisbet AJ, Xu MJ, Zhou DH, Zhao GH, et al. Characterization of *Trichuris trichiura* from humans and T. *suis* from pigs in China using internal transcribed spacers of nuclear ribosomal DNA. Journal of Helminthology. 2014;**88**(1):64-68

[14] Nissen S, Al-Jubury A, Hansen TV, Olsen A, Christensen H, Thamsborg SM, et al. Genetic analysis of *Trichuris suis* and *Trichuris trichiura* recovered from humans and pigs in a sympatric setting in Uganda. Veterinary Parasitology. 2012;**188**(1-2):68-77

[15] Nadler SA, DE LEÓN GP. Integrating molecular and morphological approaches for characterizing parasite cryptic species: Implications for parasitology. Parasitology. 2011;**138**(13):1688-1709

[16] Hawash MB, Andersen LO, Gasser RB, Stensvold CR, Nejsum P. Mitochondrial genome analyses suggest multiple *Trichuris* species in humans, baboons, and pigs from different geographical regions. PLoS Neglected Tropical Diseases. 2015;**9**(9):e0004059

[17] Rivero Fernández J, García Sánchez ÁM, Zurita Carrasco A, Cutillas Barrios C, Callejón FR. *Trichuris trichiura* isolated from Macaca sylvanus: Morphological, biometrical, and molecular study. BMC Veterinary Research. 2020;**16**(1):445

[18] Wang HB, Zhang HJ, Song LL, Zhu L, Chen M, Ren GJ, et al. Morphological and molecular confirmation of the validity of *Trichuris* rhinopiptheroxella in the endangered golden snub-nosed monkey (Rhinopithecus roxellana). Journal of helminthology. 2019;**93**(5):601-607

[19] Cutillas C, de Rojas M, Zurita A, Oliveros R, Callejón R. *Trichuris* colobae n. sp. (Nematoda: Trichuridae), a new species of *Trichuris* from Colobus guereza kikuyensis. Parasitology research. 2014;**113**(7):2725-2732

[20] Callejón R, Halajian A, Cutillas C. Description of a new species, *Trichuris* ursinus n. sp. (Nematoda: Trichuridae) from Papio ursinus Keer, 1792 from South Africa. Infection, Genetics, and Evolution. 2017;**51**:182-193

[21] Araujo A, Reinhard KJ, Ferreira LF, Gardner SL. Parasites as probes for prehistoric human migrations? Trends in parasitology. 2008;**24**(3):112-115

[22] Fahmy MA. An investigation on the life cycle of *Trichuris muris*. Parasitology. 1954;**44**(1-2):50-57

[23] Davaine CJ. Recherches sur le developpement et la propagation du Trichocephale de 1'Homme et de l'Ascaride lombricoide. Comp. rends. Acad. sc., Paris, 46: 1217-1219. 1863.-Nouvelles recherches sur le developpement et la propagation de l'Ascaride lombricoide et du Trichocephale de l'Homme. Compt. rends. Soc. biol., Paris. 1858;**3**:261-265

[24] Panesar TS. The moulting pattern in *Trichuris muris* (Nematoda: Trichuroidea). Canadian Journal of zoology. 1989;**67**(9):2340-2343

[25] Nejsum P, Betson M, Bendall RP, Thamsborg SM, Stothard JR. Assessing the zoonotic potential of Ascaris suum and *Trichuris suis*: Looking to the future from an analysis of the past. Journal of Helminthology. 2012;**86**:148-155

[26] Liu GH, Zhou W, Nisbet AJ, Xu MJ, Zhou DH, Zhao GH, et al. Characterization of *Trichuris trichiura* from humans and T. *suis* from pigs in China using internal transcribed spacers of nuclear ribosomal DNA. Journal of Helminthology. 2014;**88**:64-68

[27] Arizono N, Yamada M, Tegoshi T, Onishi K. Molecular identification of Oesophagostomum and *Trichuris* eggs isolated from wild Japanese macaques. The Korean Journal of Parasitology. 2012;**50**:253-257

[28] Gillespie TR, Lonsdorf EV, Canfield EP, Meyer DJ, Nadler Y, Raphael J, et al. Demographic and ecological effects on patterns of parasitism in eastern chimpanzees (Pan troglodytes schweinfurthii) in Gombe National Park, Tanzania. American Journal of Physical Anthropology. 2010;**143**:534-544

[29] Kooriyama T, Hasegawa H, Shimozuru M, Tsubota T, Nishida T, Iwaki T. Parasitology of five primates in the Mahale Mountains National Park Tanzania. Primates. 2012;**53**:365-375

[30] World Health Organization. Helminth Control in School-Age Children. Geneva: A guide for managers of control programs; 2011

[31] Uniting to Combat Neglected Tropical Diseases. Delivering on promises and driving progress. 2014

[32] Geerts S, Gryseels B. Anthelmintic resistance in human helminths: a review. Tropical Medicine & International Health. 2001;**6**:915-921

[33] Keiser J, Utzinger J. Efficacy of current drugs against soil-transmitted helminth infections: Systematic review and meta-analysis. Journal of the American Medical Association. 2008;**299**:1937-1948

[34] Kaplan RM, Vidyashankar AN. An inconvenient truth: Global worming and anthelmintic resistance. Veterinary Parasitology. 2012;**186**:70-78

[35] Sargison ND. Pharmaceutical treatments of gastrointestinal nematode infections of sheep—Future of anthelmintic drugs. Veterinary Parasitology. 2012;**189**:79-84

[36] Sutherland IA, Leathwick DM. Anthelmintic resistance in nematode parasites of cattle: a global issue? Trends in Parasitology. 2011;**27**:176-181

[37] Matthews J. Anthelmintic resistance in equine nematodes. International Journal for Parasitology: Drugs and Drug Resistance. 2014;**4**:310-315

[38] Kwa MSG, Veenstra JG, Roos MH. Benzimidazole resistance in Haemonchus contortus is correlated with a conserved mutation at amino acid 200 in beta-tubulin isotype 1. Molecular and Biochemical Parasitology. 1994;**63**:299-303

[39] Mottier M, Prichard RK. Genetic analysis of a relationship between macrocyclic lactone and benzimidazole anthelmintic selection on Haemonchus contortus. Pharmacogenetics and Genomics. 2008;**18**:129-140

[40] Bundy DA, Cooper ES. *Trichuris* and trichuriasis in humans. Advances in parasitology. 1989;**28**:107-173

[41] Miller MJ. Studies on the life history of Trichocephalus *vulpis*, the whipworm of dogs. Canadian Journal of Research. 1947;**25**(1):1-1

[42] Lee TD, Wright KA. The morphology of the attachment and probable feeding site of the nematode *Trichuris muris* (Schrank, 1788) Hall, 1916. Canadian Journal of Zoology. 1978;**56**(9):1889-1905

[43] Pawlowski ZS, Arfaa F, Warren KS, Mahmoud AA. Tropical and Geographical Medicine. McGraw-Hill; 1990. pp. 458-473

[44] World Health Organization. Diagnostic Techniques for Intestinal Parasitic Infections (IPI Applicable to Primary Health Care) PHC Services. World Health Organization; 1985. Available from: https://apps.who.int/iris/handle/10665/59767

[45] Gilman RH, Chong YH, Davis C, Greenberg B, Virik HK, Dixon HB. The adverse consequences of heavy *Trichuris* infection. Transactions of the Royal Society of Tropical Medicine and Hygiene. 1983;**77**(4):432-438

[46] Needham CS, Lillywhite JE, Beasley NM, Didier JM, Kihamia CM, Bundy DA. Potential for diagnosis of intestinal nematode infections through antibody detection in saliva. Transactions of the Royal Society of Tropical Medicine and Hygiene. 1996;**90**(5):526-530

[47] Traversa D. Are we paying too much attention to cardio-pulmonary

nematodes and neglecting old-fashioned worms like *Trichuris vulpis*? Parasites & Vectors. 2011;**4**:32

[48] Yoshikawa H, Yamada M, Matsumoto Y, Yoshida Y. Variations in egg size of *Trichuris trichiura*. Parasitology Research. 1989;**75**:649-654

[49] Areekul P, Putaporntip C, Pattanawong U, Sitthicharoenchai P, Jongwutiwes S. *Trichuris vulpis* and T. *trichiura* infections among schoolchildren of a rural community in northwestern Thailand: The possible role of dogs in disease transmission. Asian Biomed. 2010;**4**:49-60

[50] Meekums H, Hawash MB, Sparks AM, Oviedo Y, Sandoval C, Chico ME, et al. A genetic analysis of *Trichuris trichiura* and *Trichuris suis* from Ecuador. Parasites & Vectors. 2015;**8**:168 First phylogenetic comparison of human *Trichuris* from Asia and South America

[51] Liu GH, Gasser RB, Su A, Nejsum P, Peng L, Lin RQ, et al. Clear genetic distinctiveness between human- and pig-derived *Trichuris* based on analyses of mitochondrial datasets. PLoS Neglected Tropical Diseases. 2012;**6**:e1539 Complete mitochondrial genomes of T. *trichiura* and T. *suis* show clear genetic distinctiveness and provide strong support for the hypothesis that *Trichuris* in humans and pigs represents separate species

[52] World Health Organization. Accelerating Work to Overcome the Global Impact of Neglected Tropical Diseases—a Roadmap for Implementation. Executive summary. Geneva: World Health Organization; 2012

[53] World Health Organization. Preventive Chemotherapy in Human Helminthiasis. Coordinated Use of Anthelminthic Drugs in Control Interventions: a Manual for Health Professionals and Program Managers. World Health Organization; 2006. Available from: https://apps.who.int/iris/handle/10665/43545

[54] Bethony J, Brooker S, Albonico M, Geiger SM, Loukas A, Hotez PJ. Soil-transmitted helminth infections: Ascaris, *Trichuris*, and hookworm. Lancet. 2006;**367**:1521-1532

[55] Olsen A, Namwanje H, Nejsum P, Roepstorff A, Thamsborg SM. Albendazole and mebendazole have low efficacy against *Trichuris trichiura* in school-age children in Kabale District, Uganda. Transactions of the Royal Society of Tropical Medicine and Hygiene. 2009;**103**:443-446

[56] Silvestre A, Cabaret J. Mutation in position 167 of isotype 1 beta-tubulin gene of Trichostrongylid nematodes: Role in benzimidazole resistance? Molecular and Biochemical Parasitology. 2002;**120**:297-300

[57] Bennett AB, Anderson TJC, Barker GC, Michael E, Bundy DAP. Sequence variation in the *Trichuris trichiura* β-tubulin locus: Implications for the development of benzimidazole resistance. International Journal for Parasitology. 2002;**32**:1519-1528

[58] Diawara A, Drake LJ, Suswillo RR, Kihara J, Bundy DAP, Scott ME, et al. Assays to detect beta-tubulin codon 200 polymorphism in *Trichuris trichiura* and Ascaris lumbricoides. PLoS Neglected Tropical Diseases. 2009;**3**:e397

[59] Diawara A, Halpenny CM, Churcher TS, Mwandawiro C, Kihara J, Kaplan RM, et al. Association between response to albendazole treatment and β-tubulin genotype frequencies in soil-transmitted helminths. PLoS Neglected Tropical Diseases. 2013;**7**:e2247 An increase in the frequency of alleles

associated with resistance was observed in T. *trichiura* isolates following albendazole treatment

[60] Hansen TVA, Nejsum P, Olsen A, Thamsborg SM. Genetic variation in codons 167, 198, and 200 of the beta-tubulin gene in whipworms (*Trichuris* spp.) from a range of domestic animals and wildlife. Veterinary Parasitology. 2013;**193**:141-149

[61] Hansen TV, Thamsborg SM, Olsen A, Prichard RK, Nejsum P. Genetic variations in the beta-tubulin gene and the internal transcribed spacer 2 region of *Trichuris* species from man and baboons. Parasites & Vectors. 2013;**6**:236

[62] Geary T, Blair K, Ho N, Sims S, Thompson D. Biological functions of nematode surfaces. In: Boothroyd J, Komuniecki R, editors. Mol. Approaches to Parasitol. New York: Wiley-Liss; 1995. pp. 57-76

[63] Mottier L, Alvarez L, Ceballos L, Lanusse C. Drug transport mechanisms in helminth parasites: Passive diffusion of benzimidazole anthelmintics. Experimental Parasitology. 2006;**113**:49-57

[64] Helbæk H. Tollund mandens sidste måltid. Aarbøger Nord. Oldkynd. og Hist. Kongelige Nordiske Oldskriftsselskab. 1950;**50**:311-341

[65] Rácz SE, De Aráujo EP, Jensen E, Mostek C, Morrow JJ, Van Hove ML, et al. Parasitology in an archaeological context: Analysis of medieval burials in Nivelles Belgium. Journal of Archaeological Science. 2014;**53**:304-315

[66] Loreille O, Roumat E, Verneau O, Bouchet F, Hänni C. Ancient DNA from Ascaris: Extraction amplification and sequences from eggs collected in coprolites. International Journal for Parasitology. 2001;**31**:1101-1106

[67] Oh CS, Seo M, Chai JY, Lee SJ, Kim MJ, Park JB, et al. Amplification and sequencing of *Trichuris trichiura* ancient DNA extracted from archaeological sediments. Journal of Archaeological Science. 2010;**37**:1269-1273

[68] Lv Z, Wu Z, Zhang L, Ji P, Cai Y, Luo S, et al. Genome mining offers a new starting point for parasitology research. Parasitology Research. 2015;**114**:399-409

[69] Foth BJ, Tsai IJ, Reid AJ, Bancroft AJ, Nichol S, Tracey A, et al. Whipworm genome and dual-species transcriptome analyses provide molecular insights into an intimate host-parasite interaction. Nature Genetics. 2014;**46**:693-700. Publication describing the Genome of T. trichiura and the Genome and transcriptome of T. *muris* at various life stages and in particular parasite body parts. Immunomodulator mechanisms are identified along with new potential drug targets against trichuriasis

[70] Jex AR, Nejsum P, Schwarz EM, Hu L, Young ND, Hall RS, et al. Genome and transcriptome of the porcinewhipworm *Trichuris suis*. Nature Genetics. 2014;**46**:701-706. Publication describing the male and female genome T. *suis* and the transcriptome of the two sexes, body parts, and different life stages. The protein-encoding gene set is presented along with molecules of importance for host-parasite interaction, as well as the role of small non-coding RNAs in gene regulation

[71] Agüero F, Al-Lazikani B, Aslett M, Berriman M, Buckner FS, Campbell RK, et al. Genomic-scale prioritization of drug targets: The TDR targets database. Nature Reviews. Drug Discovery. 2008;7:900-907

[72] Britton C, Winter AD, Gillan V, Devaney E. MicroRNAs of parasitic helminths—Identification,

characterization, and potential as drug targets. International Journal for Parasitology: Drugs and Drug Resistance. 2014;**4**:85-94

[73] Allentoft ME, Sikora M, Sjögren K-G, Rasmussen S, Rasmussen M, Stenderup J, et al. Population genomics of bronze age Eurasia. Nature. 2015;**522**:167-172

[74] Cruz K, Marcilla A, Kelly P, Vandenplas M, Osuna A, Trelis M. *Trichuris trichiura* egg extract proteome reveals potential diagnostic targets and immunomodulators. PLoS Neglected Tropical Diseases. 2021;**15**(3):e0009221

[75] Dey SS, Kester L, Spanjaard B, Van A. Integrated genome and transcriptome sequencing from the same cell. Nature Biotechnology. 2014;**33**:285-289

[76] Carlsgart J, Roepstorff A, Nejsum P. Multiplex PCR on single unembryonated Ascaris (roundworm) eggs. Parasitology Research. 2009;**104**:939-943

[77] Holroyd N, Sanchez-Flores a. Producing parasitic helminth reference and draft genomes at the Wellcome Trust sanger institute. Parasite Immunology. 2012;**34**:100-107

[78] Vejzagić N, Thamsborg SM, Kringel H, Roepstorff A, Bruun JM, Kapel CMO. In vitro hatching of *Trichuris suis* eggs. Parasitology Research. 2015;**114**:2705-2714

[79] Buck A, Coakley G, Simbari F, McSorley H, Quintana J, Le Bihan T, et al. Exosomes secreted by nematode parasites transfer small RNAs to mammalian cells and modulate innate immunity. Nature Communications. 2014;**5**:5488

[80] Hansen EP, Kringel H, Williams AR, Nejsum P. Secretion of RNA-containing extracellular vesicles by the porcine whipworm, *Trichuris suis*. The Journal of Parasitology. 2015;**101**:336-340

[81] RasmussenM ASL, Waters MR, Skoglund P, DeGiorgio M, Stafford TW, et al. The genome of a late Pleistocene human from a Clovis burial site in western Montana. Nature. 2014;**506**:225-229

[82] Watts MR, James G, Sultana Y, Ginn AN, Outhred AC, Kong F, et al. A loop-mediated isothermal amplification (LAMP) assay for Strongyloides stercoralis in stool that uses a visual detection method with SYTO-82 fluorescent dye. The American Journal of Tropical Medicine and Hygiene. 2014;**90**:306-311

[83] Le TH, Nguyen NTB, Truong NH, Van De N. Development of mitochondrial loop-mediated isothermal amplification for detection of the small liver fluke Opisthorchis viverrini (opisthorchiidae; Trematoda; Platyhelminthes). Journal of Clinical Microbiology. 2012;**50**:1178-1184

[84] Rand KH, Tremblay EE, Hoidal M, Fisher LB, Grau KR, Karst SM. Multiplex gastrointestinal pathogen panels: Implications for infection control. Diagnostic Microbiology and Infectious Disease. 2015;**82**:154-157